Love it, double love it. *101 Things You Should Know About Breast Cancer* is a quality work that is welcoming to all readers and affirming for so many. I will recommend it to every breast cancer survivor and their family members, because it is a useable, workable manual for people who need to get up to speed quickly and become informed in order to obtain their best outcomes. Pam's insights of her personal journey are validating and inspiring.

Sharon M. Bigelow, RN, MSN, ANP-BC, AOCNP
Oncology nurse practitioner (30 years)
Founder and Chief Executive Officer, NavigateCancer Foundation
(sole provider of clinical navigation services for LIVE**STRONG**)

Through her book, *101 Things You Should Know About Breast Cancer,* Pam Schmid brings clarity and common sense to the most important issues surrounding breast cancer today, from the perspective of patient and educator.

Wendie Berg, MD, PhD, FACR
Diagnostic radiologist specializing in breast imaging
Internationally renowned radiology researcher
2010 Most Influential Radiology Researcher, voted by peers on AuntMinnie.com
Professor of Radiology, University of Pittsburgh School of Medicine

101 Things You Should Know About Breast Cancer is beautifully written, informative, moving, and very accessible. This book is an extremely valuable guide for women. Pam's perspectives and thoughts are valuable for advocates and physicians as well.

Victoria L. Seewaldt, MD
Professor of Medical Oncology, Duke University
Internationally recognized breast cancer researcher
Director, Breast Cancer Prevention Program,
Women's Wellness Clinic at Duke University Medical Center

Despite all of the awareness and publicity centered on breast cancer, the reality is that most women who are newly diagnosed with the disease feel blindsided, scared, and paralyzed by their diagnosis and by the sheer volume of information that is available. In *101 Things You Should Know About Breast Cancer*, Pam obtains the perfect balance between up-to-date medical information and personal experience and advice. She has been able to cover the complex fields of risk assessment, diagnosis, treatment, and survivorship in an accurate and concise way, and her unique perspective as a fitness and healthcare professional makes for a very engaging read. This book is an invaluable resource for women newly diagnosed with breast cancer, their friends and loved ones, and physicians and other healthcare professionals who treat patients with breast cancer.

Deanna J. Attai, MD, FACS
Breast Surgeon, Center for Breast Care, Inc. (CA)

D1318683

I receive emails nearly daily from cancer survivors frustrated by the gap between the research on exercise for cancer survivors and the availability of patient-friendly sources to guide survivors to take an active role in promoting their own wellness and recovery. So I was thrilled when I heard that Pam Schmid was writing *101 Things You Should Know About Breast Cancer*. Now that I've read it, I'm happy to say I have an outstanding resource to which I can point survivors when I receive those frustrated emails!

Kathryn Schmitz, PhD, MPH, FACSM
Associate Professor, University of Pennsylvania School of Medicine
Lead investigator, Physical Activity and Lymphedema (PAL) trial
Expert panelist, YMCA/Lance Armstrong Foundation Cancer Survivorship Collaborative
Lead author, Roundtable on Exercise for Cancer Survivors

Pam Schmid's book, *101 Things You Should Know About Breast Cancer,* provides heartfelt, evidence-based information that clarifies questions and soothes the soul. As a breast cancer survivor, professor, researcher, and clinician, I look forward to sharing these pearls of wisdom with others. Pam pours her heart and passion into this book, and we are blessed to have it.

Mary Lou Galantino, PT, PhD, MSCE
Professor of Physical Therapy, The Richard Stockton College of New Jersey
Adjunct Research Scholar, University of Pennsylvania School of Medicine

101 Things You Should Know About Breast Cancer is remarkable! When you learn that you or a loved one has cancer, life suddenly stands still, questions surface, and reassurance is needed. Within the pages of this book, Pam provides a guiding light with her voice and intermingling of personal experience. She gives courage to a fearful mind, rescues the reader who is lost, and brings hope to the hopeless. Pam has touched my life and journey with cancer in a profound and powerful way, and now, with her incredible words of wisdom in print, she will do the same for you. Everyone, regardless of how cancer has touched their lives, should read this masterpiece.

Suzanne Lindley, MSW
Cancer survivor
Cofounder, YES! Beat Liver Tumors
LIVE**STRONG** Leader

Just as *What to Expect When You're Expecting* is a must own for pregnant couples, *101 Things You Should Know About Breast Cancer* is a must have for anyone diagnosed with breast cancer or anyone who knows someone diagnosed. Pam is open and honest about her experience, and her passion leaps from the pages. She provides information to help take away some of the unknowns, which will help take away some of the fear for those embarking on their own journey. Pam provides facts and doable tips to help navigate the journey and maintain energy. You will be informed, in control, and empowered when you finish this book.

Julie Schwartz, MS, RD, LD
ACSM Health Fitness Specialist
Certified and licensed corporate wellness coach
Owner, NutriWell Coaching

101 THINGS

YOU SHOULD KNOW
ABOUT BREAST CANCER

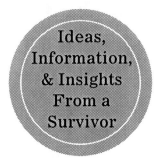

Ideas,
Information,
& Insights
From a
Survivor

Pam Schmid

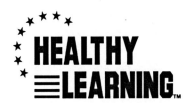

HEALTHY
LEARNING™

ISBN: 978-1-60679-190-5
Library of Congress Control Number: 2011937868
Cover design: Emily Uhland, S&A Cherokee
Cover photos: Jonathan Fredin, S&A Cherokee
Book layout: Studio J Art & Design

Healthy Learning
P.O. Box 1828
Monterey, CA 93942
www.healthylearning.com

Dedication

To my loving husband, friend, and partner, Jerry, who has supported me without end, I love you.

And—

My dear friend, Jean, who is with the angels playing joyfully, and looking down with a smile right now.

Acknowledgments

The list of people to thank is almost endless, as every person and experience have all contributed to the words on these pages, from being part of a support group for my friend, Jean, before cancer, to the health care team that supported me during treatment, to the experiences and people that have touched my life up to this very day.

The starting place of thanks go to Danielle Stanfield, close friend and founding editor of *Cary Magazine* who encouraged me to share my story early in my diagnosis and who put me on the cover, bringing interest and response that solidified the need for me to keep talking. Thank you for believing in me and for your vision and support of my efforts, your dedication to excellence and connecting to readers is a gift. From that issue to this day, *Cary Magazine* has supported me in sharing my story through reprints and help with the concept, photography, and graphics for the cover of this book, and I am forever grateful. A special thanks goes to Jonathan Fredin, photographer. You are an authentic gem; your passion, compassion, patience, and love for your work and your subjects are second to none, as is the quality of your work. Thank you to graphic designer and now editor, Emily Uhland, for helping our team with a great cover design.

I am indebted to Dr. Wendie Berg, MD, PhD, a renowned and internationally recognized radiologist who embraced my early questions about breast density and supported my advocacy and education efforts early on to teach women through speaking and a special website (www.knowyourdensity.com), reviewing both for content and accuracy. Your endless support and review for this book and its content will never be forgotten. I have been blessed and honored to know you, seeing first-hand your passion as a scientist, clinician, and educator wanting the best for women everywhere. Your award of Most Influential Radiology Researcher of the Year in 2010 by your peers validated what I knew from the moment we first spoke—that your dedication and work in finding the best methods for early detection for breast cancer are unmatched.

Sharon Bigelow, RN, MSN, ANP-BC, AOCNP, co-founder of Navigate Cancer Foundation, the world is a better place because you are here. Your passion for helping survivors and their families—including mine—is a gift. Thank you for your detailed review of every word I shared on these pages. Having someone with your experience and background review my words was invaluable. Your honesty, love, and heartfelt words gave me the strength to keep going.

To Lee Wilke, my breast surgeon and friend, thank you for your skill, intelligence, kindness, patience, and appreciation for me as an individual and my need to know in the early months of my diagnosis. I'll never forget the hours you took in counseling me through some tough conversations and the confidence you have had in me along the way. Thank you for your support with the book and your contribution to my knowledge over the years. Duke is missing a shining star, but Wisconsin is lucky to have your light.

Thanks to the team of doctors and nurses who put up with my endless questions and need to understand. They have led to a book! To my oncologist, Kelly Marcom, your thoughtful manner, empathy, compassion, and understanding made my journey easier. To Leonard Prosnitz, my radiation oncologist, thank you for your wisdom in helping me make some difficult decisions and pushing me at the right time and place. To my plastic reconstruction surgeon, Laura Gunn, your kindness gave me hope. Felicia Cofield, triage nurse extraordinaire, I couldn't have managed chemotherapy without your loving and proactive support. I will never forget you. To Kim Camp, the nurse who helped me on that first scary day of chemo, God blessed me with you that day.

To Dr. Victoria Seewaldt, Duke breast cancer researcher extraordinaire, you are a blessing and gift to womankind for your passion, intelligence, empathy, compassion, dedication, and love for the work you do and the women in the world you serve. Thank you for your confidence, support, and review of pertinent sections of this book for me.

To Lee Jones, PhD, scientific director for the Duke Center for Cancer Survivorship, your articulate passion and curiosity about the impact of exercise on tumor cells and the impact of exercise for cancer survivors is inspiring. I am blessed to know you. Thank you for the many hours of education over the years and taking time to review key sections in the book for me. Thank you to Kate Wolin, PhD, and Katie Schmitz, PhD (both ACSM fellows) for your review and incredible work in the field of cancer and exercise.

Thank you to Julie Lanford, MPH, RD, CSO, LDN, for reviewing the nutrition sections for accuracy and content. You are one of the best in the country. Many thanks to Julie Schwartz, MS, RD, CSSD, LD, ACSM-HFS, CWC, and friend for taking time to review the exercise and nutrition portions as well. I am blessed to know you and call you a friend. To Idelle Davidson, award-winning journalist and cancer survivor, thank you for your review and your book around chemo-brain. It is real.

Thank you to my incredible cancer survivor friends, who inspire me daily and for some of whom I was able to share a part of your stories, Susan Helmrich, PhD, wellness coach and three-time cancer survivor; Heidi Duskey, wellness coach and breast cancer survivor; and Suzanne Lindley, MSW, Stage IV colon cancer survivor, international cancer advocate, close friend, and teacher to the world. Whether your story was here or not, please know I am honored to know and love you. Thank you to Judy Byke, MSW and Mary Lou Galantino, PT, PhD, inspiring survivor friends for reviewing portions of the book from a survivor's point of view.

And more thanks to Dr. Galantino for finding me and wanting to collect data around my work. Without you, I would never have ventured into the research waters. The experience of being a co-investigator raised my level of understanding for the broader scope and impact to survivors through the entire process from IRBs (research boards) to the final published paper. Your beautiful spirit made the hard work bearable. Your friendship and love have brightened my world.

Thank you to Regina Heroux, RN, MS, OCN, for your years of support with our friend Jean to your support of me now, teaching and working with me as a co-chair about the world of cancer, and reviewing my words here.

To the experts from whom I have sought knowledge over the years, thank you for your patience and willingness to teach me. In particular, thank you Wendy Demark-Wahnefried, PhD, RD, for the words of wisdom and expertise before my treatment and the many answers to my questions around nutrition, exercise, and body composition over the years.

Thank you to all the Duke Survivorship researchers, clinicians, and program staff who put up with my questions, observations, opinions, and annoying passion the years I sat in on weekly meetings, strategic planning, or other focus groups. Thank you to Tina Piccirilli, the director for the Duke Center for Cancer Survivorship for believing in my programs and willingness to write a grant together. I have been grateful for your support.

Serious appreciation and thanks go to the inventors of the laptop computer, as I was able to move about my house and porches to write in the space I needed, in order to be inspired. I don't think I could have sat in one place for two years writing!

To all my friends and family who supported me with words, deeds, prayer, and love, you saw me through many ups and downs from treatment through the final words on these pages, and I am filled with gratitude. To Robin Burch, your wanting to be with me on the first day of chemo to help me through it, flying from Texas to be with me was a gift I'll never forget. Your continued love and friendship from college to this day is more than anyone could ever hope for. Kristen Dill, your understanding, friendship, and love have seen me through treatment and beyond. Thanks for being the sounding board I needed through the completion of this book. Ann Wetmore, your kind voice on the other end of the line was a precious gift during treatment. You showed me how to love someone through pain. To Jean's support group, she said we would need each other when she was gone, and she was right. I am grateful.

I would not have had the support of the previously mentioned people had I not known Jean Pendergraft. From the age of 16, I knew her as a mother of a boyfriend, and we stayed friends over the years. After her diagnosis of Stage IV breast cancer, we ended up moving back into the area and became much closer as I supported her and took her to treatments. Jean, you taught me so much about appreciating the little things in life and how to find joy in spite of difficult circumstances. Your spirit is with me, and I miss you.

To mom and dad, where would I have been without your love and support? Thank you for being proud, believing in me, and keeping me going when I didn't think I could. I am so lucky and proud to have you both as parents.

To my little sister, Patti, your unending love and belief that your big sister can do anything makes me smile. I love you.

To my sons, Dustin and Jeremy, and my daughter-in-law Caroline, I love you all more than life itself. Thank you for being by my side through my journey of breast cancer and for making me the proudest mom ever. All I've ever needed is to be your mom. I'm so lucky.

I could never have done this book without the love of my life and extreme support of my sweet husband, Jerry. You have endured and supported my passion for making a difference in the cancer world with very little, if any, income. I know you thought that this book would never come to an end, and neither did I. Two years of what we thought would be one! Finally, my love, it is here!

Foreword

In today's data-driven world, you can find many books and websites that provide accurate and helpful information about breast cancer—for patients, their loved ones, and health care providers. I look forward to the day when there won't be a need for books and online resources like these, when patients and families won't have to experience tough treatments, and when women won't die of this disease. Pam Schmid's book, *101 Things You Should Know About Breast Cancer*, is, however, a unique addition to this library of information in that it provides a concise overview of the complexities of the disease with a guide through the very human experience of breast cancer. From the moment of her own breast cancer diagnosis in 2004, Pam started speaking and writing about the disease and its treatments, wanting to help others either understand the importance of early detection or make life easier for those experiencing cancer. In this book, she puts together this wealth of personal and scientific knowledge to educate and guide others who now face this diagnosis.

Breast cancer, like people, has varied personalities and can function differently, just like people do, despite similar circumstances. Pam simply defines this important fact in her book and highlights the importance of understanding your or your loved one's own type of breast cancer. In an ideal world, we will have personalized therapies for each patient's individual breast cancer. Though progress is never as rapid as we would like, we've come a long way in the past 50 years in treating this disease. In 1882, Dr. William Halsted pioneered the Halsted Mastectomy, which radically removed the breast, lymph nodes, and muscles of the chest wall. The 130 years since have seen a multitude of changes, including "more" minimally invasive types of surgery and radiation. An explosion in "cancer drugs," holds the most promise for personalizing cancer care. It is likely that breast cancer patients in the future will be advised to take a combination of drugs that are personalized for their cancer, just like exercises (which Pam strongly recommends) that target different muscles, work best for maximizing a person's overall strength and fitness.

We have also made progress and had a steady decline in breast cancer mortality because of the strong support from patients and physicians for cancer clinical trials. It was through well-planned clinical trials in the 1960s that the lumpectomy was found to be equivalent to mastectomy for women with early stage breast cancer, and though Pam needed a mastectomy for her treatment, more and more women are eligible for this minimally invasive approach to breast cancer treatment. Clinical trials are just as important today as they were in the 1960s, providing the ability for us to determine the best personalized therapies.

As a breast cancer surgeon, I am humbled by the people I have the immense privilege to take care of every day. Pam Schmid is one of those amazing individuals. Since the moment I met her in my office at Duke University Health System in 2004, I knew she would be the one to reach out to teach others about the befores and afters of cancer. In this book, she has put together a wonderful array of facts, hints, suggestions, and very important life lessons so others can "profit" from her quest to understand cancer. She has emphasized most eloquently the importance of human wellness in the cancer struggle. Though you may still face a cancer, like Pam did, you can face it with fortitude, like she did, because you thought about how to treat your body with dignity.

To the many women, their friends, physicians, or family members who read this book, please enjoy the teachings, the simple messages, and the heartfelt strength that are entwined within its pages.

Lee Gravatt Wilke, MD
Director, UW Health Breast Center
Associate Professor of Surgery, University of Wisconsin-Madison

Contents

Preface

From the first day I was diagnosed with breast cancer, I was like an investigator on a hard case, asking questions and recording my thoughts as if my life depended on it. One could argue it did, but I wanted to be sure I knew what I needed to know to do all the right things. Information was a comfort to me mainly because it helped me feel more in control of the chaos I was feeling inside. I wanted to know every last detail about all the things that might impact my mortality and quality of life, positively or negatively.

When Jim Peterson at Healthy Learning first asked me to consider writing this book, I was ambivalent mostly because of the wealth of information that already existed in the form of books, websites, and various other media.

But when I thought about the opportunity to share some of the unique experiences and information that I have gathered as a result of my investigative nature and the experts I've been able to learn from, I decided that it might be an opportunity to share the hard-earned lessons and perspectives I've gained.

Though I am not a medical expert, I have been fortunate to get to know many of those who are and who have been generously teaching me over the past seven years. From the first week of my diagnosis, where I was attending an American College of Sports Medicine conference, learning from a Harvard breast surgeon and survivor about the physical challenges breast cancer survivors face during and after treatment, to learning over the years from internationally respected researchers and experts in the areas of early detection, nutrition, exercise, survivorship, psychosocial issues, and more.

My curiosity and passion for knowledge was what helped comfort and guide me in the extreme decision-making involved in the complicated process of becoming a patient and cancer survivor. I spent hours delving through volumes of information to know what decisions to make and what questions to ask. Sorting through the mountain of information, once again, proved to be quite overwhelming. My hope is that it has been translated simply yet still be valuable and practical.

Through the early months of diagnosis, I talked into a tape recorder, usually on my way to and from appointments, to capture all my unfiltered thoughts about what was happening. I was in a whirlwind, and it was hard to know if I was coming or going some times. Listening to those tapes again after seven years brought me back to the pain and shock of those early days, but also helped me remember the precious gift of kindness and humanity I experienced. It's those recordings that reminded me of what was important to address in the book.

My area of expertise in writing has been, first and foremost, that of a breast cancer survivor. There's nothing like going through a mastectomy and reconstruction, chemotherapy, radiation, and its after effects to teach you about having breast cancer. Being immersed as a "patient" will teach you things you never expected to learn.

And being around and learning from other cancer survivors (not just breast) through my advocacy work has not only humbled me, but it taught me that we are more alike than not, and that "survivorship" means we all share a commonality, appreciating each new day that comes.

My years of work in health promotion and fitness prepared me to use my experience to educate and help others. How could I possibly keep this experience to myself? When I was first diagnosed, I shared my story, "Cancer Will Never Happen To Me" in a magazine I had been writing health and fitness articles for (see Appendix). The response to the story let me know how important it would be for me to continue to share and educate using my voice. And this new experience of cancer gave me a unique perspective about the challenges of living well with chronic disease, cancer, or other unexpected turns in life.

Becoming involved as a patient advocate broadened my knowledge in a way no university could have ever taught. Becoming a founding member of the Duke Patient Advocacy council taught me about the many aspects of health care from an institution's perspective. I garnered a behind-the-scenes view of the inner workings that impact a patient's experience, both good and bad. I learned about patient safety and the importance of communication. Working as co-chair for the North Carolina Comprehensive Cancer Program's Survivorship Workgroup and working on our state's cancer plan exposed me to health care providers and survivors around the state and what their various agendas and focus were. I learned from being a LIVE**STRONG**® leader and delegate at three summits, meeting survivors and advocates from around the world, and learned about the issues that were important to them. Everyone had a passion and a mission to make life better for survivors. I've learned from supporting an organization and listserv of Stage IV cancer survivors (of various types) who find treatment options that are emerging but not always talked about, the many issues they face, and their hope and determination to live *with* cancer as a chronic disease, not die from it. Then, calling on Congress with cancer advocacy organizations taught me the importance of speaking up to make a difference and not being afraid of the political process. Through my work of speaking and providing coaching services to organizations, seeing the lack of money devoted to patient well-being or programming for those services, writing grants to provide the services and observing the lack of research projects translated back into real programs for survivors, I have been informed and understand the limitations of our current health care system.

Though I learned much through my own personal experience of breast cancer and my involvement with the cancer community, there is still much to learn. It is a constantly evolving field, so what we believe today may change tomorrow. I have done my best to have vital parts of the book reviewed by the nations leading experts to make sure I am on target with my facts. I've also tried to share the personal side along with the information, so that it becomes a little more engaging instead of a sheet of facts that can become quite boring.

Remember that what we know about early detection, prevention, and treatment for the disease is always evolving. Staying current with the latest trends and research (and then discussing concerns with your physician) is of utmost importance.

Introduction

Before my own breast cancer, I wonder if I would have picked up a book like this?

"Cancer Will Never Happen To Me" was the title of an article I wrote within months of my diagnosis in 2004, and may come close to what you might be thinking right now. "It's not in my family," you might say, or "I have a very healthy lifestyle, doing all the 'right' things." The idea of cancer isn't on your radar and doesn't even seem like a remote possibility. I understand. It wasn't on mine, either.

My greatest wish is that you will continue reading through the first sections, so you can learn more about your risk and what you can do to detect cancer at its earliest stages, never finding yourself in my shoes! Stay with me.

If you've been diagnosed with cancer, I hope you will read the book in full, so you will be informed, validated, supported, empowered, inspired, hopeful, and able to share important information with those around you to better support you, make your journey easier, and help dispel misinformation and myths.

If you picked up the book to learn more about what a friend or loved one is going through, bless you. Understanding the scope of what they may be experiencing will be invaluable for them. Cancer doesn't just happen to the person who has it; it touches everyone within reach. The more you know, the more you can be a part of their healing and support.

If you are thinking about reading this book to learn more about your patients or clients who have been diagnosed, even more blessings to you. We need professionals who "get" what our experience has been.

Before 2004, breast cancer was something that happened to other, unfortunate souls. As a healthy and fit 46-year-old, I thought I was impervious to disease. After all, I had spent a career teaching people how to live healthy lives and prevent disease, *and* was walking the walk, as you will see in the book. I was never going to have to worry about breast cancer, or so I thought.

Before I was diagnosed, I knew a few things for sure: annual mammograms starting at age 40 were important and that women sometimes died of breast cancer. I knew their treatment often included surgery, chemotherapy, and radiation, but that was the extent of it. I did have some crazy ideas about people I knew who had the disease and what they had done to cause it. So much so, that I remember watching a friend who used to wash her dishes by hand with soapy water and never rinsed them, letting it drain off, thinking this might have played a role in her developing breast cancer! Secretly hypothesizing why someone *else* (or you) got cancer, is common, but I encourage you to arm yourself with information and the facts.

As you will learn, we don't have many clear answers on how and why people get breast cancer, other than the "risks" of being a woman and getting older. The majority of the time, no identifiable risk factors are present. We have much to learn.

Just being around someone who has breast cancer will not mean you understand what there is to know. Having taken a close friend with Stage IV breast cancer to chemotherapy and radiation for years, I was no wiser. In all my involvement with her, I really had no idea what she was dealing with. She didn't talk much about her challenges, and made it look easy. I had no idea of the complexity of the disease or what she was experiencing. A simple book would have helped me understand her experience more fully and perhaps helped me support her better. Two years after her death, I learned the intimate details by personal experience.

I have also learned that most women know about pink ribbons and raising money for breast cancer, but they don't know a lot about their own risk, early detection, or other important information that could save their lives. Also, women with breast cancer often don't understand the details of their very disease or who have gathered misinformation (or no information) that could cost them their lives, or at the very least, their quality of life.

There is much to learn about breast cancer. I understand that it is overwhelming, even for me. I've condensed a lot of information, shared my personal experience to bring the book alive, and broken it down into key sections to make it easier to grasp when needed. Starting with understanding risk and early detection, through diagnosis and treatment, well-being during and after treatment, how to navigate the "support" waters for yourself and others, and what survivorship is all about, it is a progression through the experience of being a cancer survivor.

Before my treatment began, I remember thinking how odd it was that I felt perfectly fine, yet there was a tumor growing inside of me. My thought was, "I am healthy and fit *with* cancer. How could that be? Here I am at 46 years old, running nearly an eight-minute mile with boundless energy, but have something growing inside of me that could potentially shorten my life!" I knew I would be healthy and fit *after* my diagnosis of cancer, if there was any way possible. But I had no idea how challenging that would be.

Therefore, I summarize some of the key pieces I have learned through my own experience and that of working with survivors in my Healthy and Fit After Cancer® program, with expanded sections around health and well-being during and after treatment.

Chapters 8 and 9 are helpful to understand a survivor's experience and what might be helpful and what might not, when it comes to support (on both sides). Every one of us is different and unique in what their needs and experiences are, but hopefully, it can bring about awareness of what might be a starting place.

I recognize that my audience will be diverse, from those who know very little about breast cancer, to experts and those living in the trenches with the disease. To the experts (including survivors), please understand that I am trying to give as much evidence-based information as possible and have had to simplify and shorten a lot of the information, not including every detail. To those who are new to breast cancer, the information presented here is just the tip of the iceberg, and it is intended to hit some of the most basic, compelling, or asked-about topics. Many of the websites I refer to are an endless source of information. For survivors, I hope that the book may shed light on subjects you may not know about, spark curiosity to learn more, and otherwise be a source of information and support to make life easier.

Throughout the book, I have shared my perspective on many of the topics as a survivor, intermingled with facts and information. People have said they like reading my personal thoughts and experiences before the sections (and some throughout). As to those personal thoughts, I'm always surprised at what people glean from the written page. I pray that my words are read with the understanding that this is *my* story and experience, and are written with the utmost respect and knowledge of stories much better and much worse, and different. I am humbled by the knowledge of others' experiences. My love and respect go out to you. I hope at least some of my words validate your experience and give you hope.

To all of you who have been touched by breast cancer, I wish you peace, love, and much hope to navigate your journey.

1

Risk, Prevention, Myths, and Other Facts: Can It Happen to You?

The first two chapters of the book contain information most people will want to know to determine if breast cancer can happen to them and what they can do to detect it early. The bottom line is that if you are a woman, you are at risk. The more you know, the more proactive you can be in catching it early, avoiding aggressive treatments, and possibly saving your life. I thought I had almost no risk, but I was wrong. Most of the time no risk factors, other than being a woman, are identifiable. At the beginning of Chapter 3: When Someone Is Diagnosed, I write more about my personal prevention efforts.

#1: Breast cancer is an uncontrolled growth of breast cells that is triggered by damage to the cells' DNA.

My first question to the doctor on the morning of my diagnosis, was *how* does breast cancer begin and why? How could this happen when I have done everything "right" to avoid it? His scientific answer was brief and simple, but summed it up: "It's basically a result of damage to your DNA … but we may not ever know exactly how or when that damage happened or what caused your breast cancer."

Our bodies are constantly producing new cells. When they become damaged, old, or we don't need them, the cells go through a normal process of cell death, called apoptosis. When this normal process of cell death doesn't happen, an uncontrolled growth of cells can occur.

A mutation or damage to the DNA is often responsible for this process to change, giving the cell the ability to keep dividing without control. Damage can occur from environmental factors (such as chemicals, UV light, and radiation), from an inability to prevent cancer (which you are born with), or from normal metabolic processes inside the cell.

#2: The statistics concerning women and breast cancer are alarming.

As you read these statistics, I encourage you to consider that each of these numbers represent a daughter, a wife, a sister, a mother, an aunt, a grandmother, or a friend in the community. The ripple effect of how it impacts our society is tremendous and touches nearly everyone.

Every two minutes, someone is diagnosed in the United States, representing an estimated 230,480 new diagnoses of invasive breast cancer each year.* Another 57,650 are diagnosed with the earliest stage 0 breast cancer, called in-situ breast cancer (meaning it hasn't spread outside the duct to other tissue). Some debate exists as to whether "in-situ" should be described as cancer or a "pre-cancer," because it is possible it may never develop into an invasive, life-threatening cancer.

About 1.3 million women will be diagnosed with breast cancer worldwide each year.

Every 69 seconds, a woman will die of this disease worldwide; nearly one a minute. Breast cancer is the leading cause of cancer death in women worldwide, with nearly

---

*These statistics are estimates from the American Cancer Society's Cancer Facts and Figures 2011.

465,000 deaths predicted in 2007, according to the Global Facts and Figures 2007 from the American Cancer Society.

Every 13 minutes, a woman will die of breast cancer in the United States. Breast cancer kills approximately 40,000 women each year in our country.

#3: Seventy-five percent of the time, no identifiable risk factors are present for women diagnosed with breast cancer.

For the majority of women diagnosed with cancer, no risk factors (family history or exposures) can be identified as the cause. Multiple scientific researchers are working on this to try to identify those women who might be at risk. This statistic is one of the most eye-opening facts because many women falsely believe they don't need to worry if they have no history of breast cancer in their family.

#4: Eighty-five percent of women who are diagnosed with breast cancer have no family history.

For women who do have a family history (about 15 percent), their risk is increased, but, even for them, it does not mean they will develop the disease.

#5: If you are a woman, you are at risk. If you are getting older, you are at risk.

The majority of breast cancer cases happen in women. It is 100 times more common in women than in men. The lifetime risk of getting breast cancer is 1 out of 8, but that is only if you live to be 80 years old.

At any given age, the following is what the likelihood would be for developing breast cancer in the next 10 years*:

- At 20 years old: 1 out of 1,760
- At 30 years old: 1 out of 229
- At 40 years old: 1 out of 69
- At 50 years old: 1 out of 42
- At 60 years old: 1 out of 29
- At 70 years old: 1 out of 27
- By age 80: 1 out of 8

*From American Cancer Society Breast Cancer Facts and Figures 2009-2010

#6: Men can get breast cancer, but they have a very low risk of developing it.

Though it is rare, men are sometimes diagnosed with breast cancer. According to the American Cancer Society, the lifetime risk of breast cancer for men is about 1 in 1,000. The most recent estimate for male breast cancer in the United States for 2011 was approximately 2,140 cases annually with 450 dying from the disease.

Men with the same stage of cancer have the same survival rates. It used to be thought that the prognosis was worse for men than for women, but women's and men's survival rates are the same. Many men who develop breast cancer are at genetic high risk due to a BRCA2 mutation: genetic counseling is usually appropriate for that man and perhaps his relatives (see #10).

#7: Breast cancer can occur in women of any age.

Certainly as women age, they are at higher risk for breast cancer, but women at any age can get breast cancer. Nearly 80 percent of all breast cancer is diagnosed in women over age 50.

The risk is lower the younger you are, but it does occur in women of all ages. Twenty percent of women diagnosed with breast cancer are in their 40s. Routine annual mammographic screening is recommended to begin at age 40 for women of average risk, but regardless of your age or when you begin annual screening, it is important to know your body and discuss anything unusual with your doctor.

The youngest known case of breast cancer in the United States occurred in 2009, in a young girl in California diagnosed when she was 10 years old. She was found to have an invasive ductal carcinoma, and was Stage IIA (see Chapter 3: When Someone Is Diagnosed). Of course, this particular instance is an extremely rare occurrence, but it illustrates the fact that women of any age should be aware of unusual changes in their breasts and have them evaluated by a trusted health care provider.

I personally have met women with breast cancer found in their 20s and many more in their 30s and 40s. However, it's important to know that most women will never develop breast cancer.

#8: Breast cancer is the leading cause of *cancer* death for women diagnosed in their 40s.

This statistic illustrates the importance of regular annual screening for women starting at age 40. Breast cancer is highly survivable when caught at early stages. It is also the leading cause of *cancer* death for women 15 to 54 years old.

#9: Using checklists or risk assessment tools can give a false sense of security about risk.

Physicians may use models to help them identify women at a *high* or *intermediate risk* so they can determine if earlier screening, additional screening, or possible early interventions should be considered.

However, because no one can accurately predict who will and who won't get breast cancer, people should use caution when looking at checklists. Risk assessment tools can help understand increased risk, but should never be used to assume *no* risk or that regular screening is not important.

In my case, I had a 98.6 percent chance of *not* getting breast cancer, according to one assessment tool predicting *five-year risk*. As you have read up until now, the majority of the time, women diagnosed with breast cancer have few, if any, risk factors.

When I completed the National Cancer Institutes Breast Cancer Risk Assessment tool, as if it were the year before I was diagnosed, I had a 1.4 percent risk of getting breast cancer in the next five years, which compares to an average woman who has a risk of 1 percent at age 46. That translated into a 98.6 percent chance that I would *not* be diagnosed with breast cancer in the near future. For any given individual, in any given year, you either do or do not have detectable breast cancer; that is, on a personal level the "risk" is essentially all or none at any given time.

> I believe that there is danger in looking at risk calculations and checklists because there is a tendency to think we are off the hook and may not be vigilant in regular screening. I did not think it was possible for me to get breast cancer. That may have led to my skipping a few years, in fact, when I might have found my cancer earlier.

Other calculations or models may be more accurate giving a 10-year or lifetime risk that might have put my risk a bit higher, but the point is that we tend to look at the checklists and believe we don't have to worry about our annual screening.

The risk assessment tool on the National Cancer Institute's website uses the Gail model, and looks at the following risks:

- Getting older
- Age at the start of menstruation (younger than 12 is higher risk)
- Age at first live birth (after 35 or never having a child is higher risk)
- Number of maternal (mother's side) first-degree relatives (mother, sisters, daughters) with breast cancer
- Number of previous breast biopsies (whether positive or negative)
- At least one breast biopsy with atypical hyperplasia

They note that other risk factors are not in the tool yet because evidence on how these factors contribute to risk is not conclusive, they did not yet have the data to include it in the model, or because they did not know whether additional factors would add useful information to the model/calculation. The Gail model is accurate for Caucasian women, but may not be as accurate for women of Hispanic, Asian, or African descent.

Some other risk factors not in the Gail model include:
- Paternal (father's side) family history
- Family history in second-degree relatives, such as aunt, grandmother, or cousin
- Family history of a male with breast cancer
- Age of diagnosis of relatives with breast cancer
- Family history or personal history of ovarian cancer
- Dense breast tissue on a mammogram
- Radiation exposure
- Age of menopause (after age 55)
- Environmental pollutants
- Use of hormone replacement therapy*
- A high-fat diet*
- Drinking alcohol*
- Low physical activity or lack of exercise*
- Obesity or high body mass index, especially weight gain after menopause*

At this time, we do not know anyone who is immune to this disease. However, you can do some things to reduce your risk of breast cancer, which are discussed in the next pages.

*Risks we can impact or do something about.

#10: A strong family history may increase the risk of having an inherited mutation in the genes and lead to breast cancer.

A strong family history may increase the risk of having an inherited mutation in genes called BRCA1 or BRCA2, but this applies to only about 2 to 5 percent of adult women in the general population.

A strong family history usually means having two or more first-degree relatives diagnosed with breast cancer, such as a mother, sister, or daughter. Second-degree relatives (aunts, nieces, or grandmothers) can be significant under certain situations as noted in the following bulleted lists. Since breast cancer in men is rare, a family history of a man with breast cancer is almost always important.

Some women may have an inherited mutation of genes connected to breast and ovarian cancer, called BRCA1 or BRCA2. Testing for the genes is done through a blood test and requires genetic counseling before and after. It is not usually done unless certain familial patterns or history are present, as noted on the National Cancer Institute website.

For women of Ashkenazi Jewish descent:
- Any first-degree relative with breast or ovarian cancer
     and
- Two second-degree relatives on the same side of the family with breast or ovarian cancer

For women who are *not* of Ashkenazi Jewish descent:
- Two first-degree relatives (mother, daughter, or sister) with breast cancer, one of whom was diagnosed at age 50 or younger
- Three or more first-degree or second-degree (grandmother or aunt) relatives with breast cancer regardless of their age at diagnosis
- A combination of first- and second-degree relatives with breast cancer and ovarian cancer (one cancer type per person)
- A first-degree relative with cancer in both breasts (bilateral breast cancer)
- A combination of two or more first- or second-degree relatives with ovarian cancer regardless of age at diagnosis
- A first- or second-degree relative with both breast *and* ovarian cancer regardless of age at diagnosis
- Breast cancer diagnosed in a male relative.

Having a known BRCA gene mutation does not mean that breast cancer will develop in that person, but it does mean that person is at an increased risk. Breast cancer is more likely to strike at a younger age in BRCA-mutation carriers, especially those with a BRCA1 mutation.

#11: Breast density is an important new risk factor.

Recent studies have shown that women who have breasts with high density have four to six times more risk for developing breast cancer than those with fatty breasts. Breast density describes the amount of glandular and connective tissue versus fatty tissue in the breast. For most women, breast density decreases with age but some women have dense breast tissue throughout their life.

Currently, the primary method for determining breast density is from a mammogram where a visual estimation of breast density is given in a report (see Chapter 2: Early Detection). If a woman has a lot of dense breast tissue, seeing a tumor on a mammogram is more difficult because tumors are white and so is dense tissue. However, mammography is still helpful for women with dense breasts because it can catch some types of early stage cancers (in-situ) or other changes seen from year to year that may indicate a need to do further imaging, such as ultrasound.

As a side note, in a recent study of 475 post-menopausal women taking estrogen and progesterone hormone treatments, a 19 percent rise in their breast density was noted which translated into 3.6 times more cases of cancer.

Breast density is not currently part of risk calculations but will most likely be added in the near future. It appears that some dense breast tissue is more "active" than others, for example showing increased background enhancement on MRI or increased metabolic activity on nuclear medicine studies. Such active dense tissue may better predict risk than just mammographically dense tissue: this is an area of ongoing research investigation. See Chapter 2: Early Detection to learn more about breast density.

#12: Preventing breast cancer is a myth.

While we can reduce risk for breast cancer, we cannot prevent it. Scientists believe we can do certain things to reduce our risk, but no sure formula for total prevention is available.

When I was diagnosed, I was in shock because I didn't know how cancer could have happened to me. I had spent a career in health promotion/disease prevention and had taken every precaution associated with lowering my risk.

The day after my diagnosis, I left for a scheduled conference with the American College of Sports Medicine. I remember passionately seeking out revered scientists, asking how someone who had done everything "right" could still develop cancer. It may sound naive, but I was frustrated and confused about all I had done to "prevent" cancer. Their answer was something we don't hear enough: "We can *reduce* risk of disease, but we cannot always prevent it."

In other words, we can stack the odds in our favor, but at this time there is no foolproof way to *prevent* breast cancer. Even prophylactic mastectomy does not completely remove the risk of breast cancer, because some small amounts of breast tissue will remain.

Even if you can't totally prevent disease, you should do all you can to reduce your risk. In the event you were diagnosed, you would be starting treatment at a higher level of health and well-being to manage the impact of treatment.

#13: You can reduce your risk for many cancers by living a healthy lifestyle.

According to the American Cancer Society, evidence is strong that poor diets, sedentary lifestyles, and carrying excess weight are linked to one third of all 550,000 cancer deaths (not just breast) each year.

The American Institute for Cancer Research offers the following evidence-based recommendations for cancer prevention:
- Be as lean as possible without becoming underweight.
- Be physically active for at least 30 minutes every day.
- Avoid sugary drinks.
- Limit consumption of energy-dense (high-calorie) foods.
- Eat a variety of vegetables, fruits, whole grains, and legumes such as beans.
- Limit consumption of red meats (such as beef, pork, and lamb), and avoid processed meats.
- If consumed at all, limit alcoholic drinks to two for men and one for women per day.
- Limit consumption of salty foods and foods processed with salt (sodium).
- Don't use supplements to protect against cancer.
- It is best for mothers to breastfeed exclusively for up to six months, and then add other liquids and foods.
- After treatment, cancer survivors should follow the recommendations for cancer prevention.
- Don't smoke or chew tobacco.

The American Cancer Society gives similar advice for lowering risk:
- Limit alcohol intake.
- Exercise regularly.
- Maintain a healthy body weight.
- Breast-feed for at least several months.
- Avoid post-menopausal hormone therapy (including what some practitioners call bio-identical or natural hormones).

> Research is accumulating around the importance of Vitamin D in reducing risk for breast cancer, but is not definitive.

You can reduce your risk of breast cancer by 40 percent by engaging in healthy habits.

The American Institute of Cancer Research believes that 40 percent of breast cancers can be prevented by six months of breastfeeding, limiting alcohol to one drink or less per day, exercising for 30 minutes five days a week, and having a normal weight.

#14: Women who exercise regularly are less likely to develop or die from breast cancer.

Exercise is one way to reduce your risk of developing cancer. Women with high aerobic fitness levels have a 55 percent lower chance of dying from breast cancer than those who are not as fit, according to research from the Aerobics Center Longitudinal Study at Cooper Clinic in Dallas, Texas. This result was after they controlled for BMI (body mass index), smoking, family history, and other risk factors. According to the NCI, exercising four or more hours a week may decrease hormone levels, which lowers breast cancer risk.

If you know my story, you might be saying, why should I bother? You did all of that, and it didn't help you! Well, I understand. But stacking the odds in your favor is what we are talking about. Additionally, we don't know if my exercising might have prevented it from coming sooner. It also allowed me to have a higher level of health when starting chemotherapy. More than anything, exercise has always improved my quality of life before and after cancer. We know that sedentary living is one of the largest risk factors for all causes of mortality or death (same Cooper Clinic study as above). I also had taken soy protein supplements in the few years before my diagnosis which may have impacted my risk (see #17).

#15: Alcohol consumption is associated with an increased risk of breast cancer.

Drinking two or more alcoholic drinks a day increases breast cancer risk one-and-a-half times over those who do not drink. In general, the level of risk increases with greater consumption. A drink is defined as 12 ounces of regular beer, 5 ounces of wine, or 1.5 ounces of 80-proof liquor.

Researchers believe there may be an association with alcohol for several reasons. Alcohol causes estrogen levels to increase, which is associated with certain types of breast cancer. Alcohol may also reduce levels of folic acid, which is involved in copying and repairing DNA. Low levels might play a role in DNA not being copied correctly when the cells divide, which can lead to cancerous growth.

For those who drink in moderation, it may be helpful to make sure folic acid is plentiful in the diet with oranges, orange juice, green leafy vegetables, or fortified cereals, according to recent research, though study results are not definitive.

The best recommendation according to the most recent research is to either not drink, or to drink occasionally, with just one drink per occasion to lower risk.

Because heart disease is a leading killer of women, it's important to mention that some research has pointed to moderate consumption of alcohol reducing the risk of heart disease. Women should discuss their individual situations and current lifestyle factors that impact overall health, such as exercising regularly, and maintaining a healthy body weight in addition to the role alcohol may play.

Interestingly, in a recent study at Kaiser Permanente of Northern California, post-menopausal women who had been diagnosed with early stage breast cancer and had a normal weight (BMI < 25) did not increase their risk of *recurrence* of breast cancer by drinking three to four drinks per week; however, overweight or obese postmenopausal women did increase their risk.

#16: Being overweight after menopause increases risk of breast cancer.

Before menopause, there does not appear to be an association with obesity and increased risk of breast cancer, but after menopause there is. After menopause, a significant source of estrogen comes from body fat. Estrogen is associated with the most common type of breast cancer, and too much circulating estrogen may stimulate breast cancer growth.

Obesity is typically defined as a BMI (body mass index) of 30 or more. The Internet provides BMI calculators with which you input height and weight to find your BMI. As noted, to reduce your risk of breast cancer, the best plan is to be as lean as possible without being underweight.

#17: Soy supplements may increase risk of breast cancer.

Research is still out on the benefits or harm of soy products as they pertain to breast cancer risk, but most scientists agree that taking soy in any way *other* than in whole forms—like tofu, edamame, or milk—may be harmful.

The most common type of breast cancer is fueled by estrogen. Soy contains isoflavones that can act like estrogen. Research is being conducted about the role soy may play in breast cancer risk. Some researchers believe it may be protective in its whole form (like tofu or soy milk), while others believe it may actually stimulate breast cancer growth in humans. Most experts agree that eating soy in its whole form in moderation is fine, but supplements with concentrated amounts should be avoided.

Though I will never know for sure what caused my cancer, I believe soy isoflavones from supplements may have played a role. Because I had reduced every possible risk remotely associated with breast cancer, this was one piece out of the ordinary. In fact, the first sentence out of my mouth to the doctor the morning of my diagnosis was about my use of soy and whether it could have caused my cancer.

I was taking a medical grade soy powder that was the equivalent of 6 cups of regular soymilk per day, for nearly two years. It was a good source of protein, and I took it for a couple of reasons I believed would be beneficial to my health. In addition, I was eating health bars that contained a lot of soy protein and drinking regular soy milk.

I share this to point out that, as Americans, we grab onto the latest news headline or claim without sometimes fully understanding the science. "If some is good, more must be better" is a belief many follow.

I would not take a supplement like that again, obviously, but I think it's also important to share how I was pulled into what I thought was credibility and safety. Aside from the claims, the descriptions about the product provided what most individuals would consider assurance of safety. The descriptions from the packaging and website included statements like, "medical grade soy," "certified isoflavone levels," "certified genetically-pure soy," "no chemical processing," "#1 doctor–recommended," "used in research trials funded by NIH clinically tested," "recommended by thousands of doctors, dietitians, and healthcare professionals," and "antioxidants equivalent to 6 cups of soymilk, and naturally concentrated." I was very careful to investigate the company before I took it, including calling the "doctor" on staff, who was a PhD, not a medical doctor (which at the time, I thought was a little misleading as a consumer). What I didn't know was that the science behind the claims was not there. "Used in research trials" does not mean that it is safe and cannot cause harm. You would have to look at what trials were performed, where they were conducted, and what the results actually were. Sometimes, the headlines do not tell the whole story.

What I know for sure, and what I have learned from nationally recognized researchers in the field of nutrition, is that concentrated sources of anything can have a medicinal effect, acting just like medication. Medications or drugs go through rigorous processes of approval before they go to market, with years of research to show what impact they may have on the human body. At this time, we do not have definitive answers regarding soy *supplements*, but most experts agree that they are not recommended.

#18: Common myths are associated with breast cancer risk.

Myth: Using antiperspirants will cause breast cancer.

No evidence has shown an association of antiperspirant use with breast cancer. Some research has looked at the relationship with parabens and aluminum-based compounds in relation to breast cancer. Parabens are found in some personal care, food, and pharmaceuticals and mimic the activity of estrogen in the body's cells. The association with aluminum is that it can cause estrogen-like effects that could possibly contribute to the growth of breast cancer cells. No study has been able to find an association between antiperspirant use and breast cancer.

Myth: Women with large breasts get breast cancer, and women with small breasts do not.

Some women believe that if they have small breasts they are less likely to develop breast cancer. No evidence suggests that smaller breasted women have less breast cancer. While a range of breast density is found with any size breasts, small breasts are more likely to be denser than larger breasts, which are more often fatty. Since dense breast tissue increases the risk of developing breast cancer *and* can mask it on mammography, smaller breasted women are, if anything, often at greater risk of developing breast cancer than women with large breasts.

I've met people who were quite convinced that having small breasts meant they were not at risk. One beautiful, well-educated woman remarked confidently to me, that because she had such incredibly small breasts, she was not at risk. She insisted that because there was not enough tissue to squeeze into a mammography machine, she was safe. Unfortunately, breast cancer does not know the difference between a large or small breast.

Myth: A low-fat diet will decrease your risk of breast cancer.

Not a lot of evidence can be found to support that a low-fat diet will decrease the risk of breast cancer. A low-fat diet may help a woman reduce her overall body fat, which can reduce a woman's risk, but eating a low-fat diet, by itself, has not been proven to reduce breast cancer risk.

Myth: Breast cancer is contagious.

Scientists know for certain that breast cancer is not spread from person to person. Though it may seem like an outrageous idea that it would be infectious in any way, women with breast cancer have often been ostracized in cultures and communities around the world, believing the women were contagious. During my treatment, I remember speaking to an eight-year survivor, who said she feared speaking about her cancer in her community. She was afraid of the ramifications from others knowing, partly because of the mistaken belief that it was something they could catch.

Myth: Wearing a bra with underwire will cause breast cancer.

No scientific evidence is available to support this idea.

Chapter References

American Cancer Society. *Breast Cancer Facts & Figures 2009-2010*. Atlanta, Ga.: American Cancer Society, Inc.

American Cancer Society. *Cancer Facts & Figures 2011*. Atlanta, Ga.: American Cancer Society, Inc.

American Cancer Society
www.cancer.org.

BreastCancer.org
www.BreastCancer.org.

National Cancer Institute
www.cancer.gov.

Susan G. Komen for the Cure
www.Komen.org.

2

Early Detection

This chapter is devoted to the things you should know about early detection of breast cancer so you can understand, partner, and be an advocate for yourself and others in detecting cancer at its earliest stages, when it is most curable. My story of early detection is intermingled throughout the chapter to bring the facts to life and further explain how the information not only played a role in my diagnosis, but how others might use it to their benefit.

#19: Breast cancer has a nearly 100 percent five-year survival rate when detected early.

For this reason, it is so important to detect breast cancer early. This statistic means that women who find and treat their breast cancer early will still be cancer-free after five years. According to the National Cancer Institute's Surveillance, Epidemiology, and End Results (SEER) database, for women diagnosed with breast cancer between 1988 and 2001, and diagnosed with Stage 0 or I, their five-year relative survival rate was nearly 100 percent.

This statistic does not include women who are diagnosed at stages II to IV. Prognosis is an individual matter, and survival rates are based on many factors. Though there is no way to know a person's individual prognosis, the higher the stage, the lower the survival rate.

In the spirit of educating and understanding the seriousness of the disease, if the cancer is not caught early, the five-year survival rates for Stages II to IV range from 86 percent to 20 percent, respectively. These numbers are only useful as a general guide because they reflect dying of all causes, don't reflect other individual factors such as age, general health, or tumor characteristics, and the data came from using drugs/treatment protocols that were used in the late 1990s. The survival rates would likely be higher if current treatment protocols were in the figures. The numbers do show that breast cancer is something we must still take very seriously, because it does take our mothers, daughters, sisters, and loved ones way too soon.

It's important to note that new treatments are becoming available that will extend lives in ways we have never seen before, allowing breast cancer to become a chronic disease. I have known many Stage IV survivors who lived well past 10 years, and one who was diagnosed at Stage IV with metastasis to the liver, but is now showing *no* evidence of the disease because of new treatments. Percentages and odds are defied every single day. Science cannot accurately predict what one individual's prognosis will be. No matter what stage disease someone has when diagnosed, there is hope.

For more information about stages, see Chapter 3: When Someone Is Diagnosed.

#20: Mammography is still the best tool available to *screen* for breast cancer.

Screening means testing for disease before any signs or symptoms are present. Though exciting new technologies are being developed for breast cancer screening, most professionals believe that mammography is the gold standard, and is not likely to change any time soon. Mammography is the only screening test that has been proven to reduce deaths due to breast cancer. Currently, ultrasound and MRI are additional imaging tools professionals use when further imaging is necessary, in addition to mammography.

Mammography can show changes in the breast often two years or more before anything can be felt. When detected early, not only is the likelihood of survival higher, but the treatment is often less invasive, which may include being able to do less extensive surgery to remove the cancer.

Mammography has proven to save lives over the last two decades, helping reduce breast cancer mortality in the United States by nearly one third. It is a breast exam that uses a non-invasive, low dose x-ray of each breast that gives the doctor a picture of the breast and helps identify changes and abnormalities from "normal." The breast is compressed between two panels to get a clear picture in several positions.

The amount of radiation received from a mammogram is less than that received from cosmic radiation during an airplane flight from New York to Los Angeles.

Many women have dense breast tissue, which makes mammography less effective, but it is still vital to have a mammogram, because it can pick up subtle changes from prior years that will alert the radiologist to do further imaging using other technologies. It is also the primary screening tool that can determine if you have dense breast tissue.

#21: Annual mammograms should begin at age 40.

Every professional organization that specializes in breast imaging and early detection, believes that women should start having an annual mammogram by age 40.

- Twenty percent of women diagnosed with breast cancer are in their 40s.
- Breast cancer is the leading cause of cancer death for women diagnosed in their 40s.

Though no technology is perfect, including mammography, it is the accepted gold standard and the best technology we have available. The most important message is that going for your annual screening appointment will allow you the best possible chance of detecting cancer early. As with any screening test, risks are involved with extra testing even if no cancer is present, and these risks are slightly greater in younger women than in older women.

Thermography should not be used as a substitute for mammography in detecting breast cancer. Thermography has not been demonstrated to have value as a screening, diagnostic, or adjunctive imaging tool for detecting breast cancer and may delay an early diagnosis. For more information read the FDA warning and statement from the ACR and SBI at www.acr.org.

#22: Mammograms should not be painful.

Women sometimes say they avoid going for their mammograms because they think they will hurt. Mammograms are no doubt uncomfortable, but should not be painful. Squeezing our breasts between two plates can be highly uncomfortable, but it is only for a few seconds. Should it be painful, make sure you let the technologist who is conducting the test know. Don't be shy. More than that, if the response to your pain is anything other than kind, apologetic, or accommodating, stop and ask for someone else.

The clinical director and radiologist of a large imaging facility told me once that a mammogram should never be painful. I was surprised to hear this, and I suggested she put little signs in all of the rooms that said, "Mammography may be uncomfortable, but it should not be painful. If it is, please let us know!"

They know that if women have a bad experience, they may not return, so it is imperative that they treat women with respect and care as they venture into this sometimes intimidating procedure.

> Keep in mind that the pain of being diagnosed in the later stages of cancer, where there may not be a cure, is much greater than any momentary pain or discomfort a woman may experience from a mammogram.

#23: Technology is not perfect in detecting breast cancer.

I start by saying this, because I believe it's important for patients and consumers to be knowledgeable regarding the early detection of breast cancer, or any disease for that matter. All of us benefit if we understand that we have amazing technologies, but there are limitations to the science as well as the human variables that include interpretation, skill, and experience of those working with the technology.

As a patient, you can help the equation of early detection when you communicate clearly about your symptoms or share other important background information, and make sure your prior breast imaging records and images are available at the time of your appointment. You help the equation when you do your part with all of the items discussed in this chapter and summarized at the end. You must take an active role and be knowledgeable about your body and the tests and procedures in which you are taking part.

The most important limitation to mammography is that of detecting cancer in women who have dense breast tissue. This is discussed fully in the rest of the chapter.

#24: Breast self-exams (BSE) are important.

Everyone agrees that knowing your body is important, and alerting your doctor if anything seems out of the ordinary or unusual for you is prudent. Some of the things to look or feel for include: puckering of your breast skin, bloody discharge from your nipple, persistently increased warmth or redness, a thickening or palpable lump, or a dramatic change in the size and shape of your breast.

I've heard various descriptions of how people felt or saw something different. One woman I spoke to talked about a "thickening" she felt. More commonly, I hear survivors, who felt what I did, describe it as a small pebble-like lump. I always remember wondering what cancer would feel like while doing a breast exam. I would feel the models at health fairs and be frustrated not really knowing or understanding what to search for. I felt all kinds of lumpiness or other things in my own breasts that I wasn't sure were normal over the years. However, the day I did feel something that turned out to be cancer, it felt very different than anything I'd ever felt before. That's precisely what I'd been told: "You'll know. It will be different."

Until the radiologist saw some changes they just wanted to watch, I didn't feel anything. Because they told me where the area was, I went home and did a breast self-exam. I felt something like a tiny pebble in my breast, which then led to a follow-up with my doctor. He didn't feel it, and told me I could see a surgeon if I was concerned, but suggested I just wait for the follow-up exam in six months. That story is continued later in this chapter.

When women hear that some major cancer organizations have backed away from teaching or recommending breast self-exams, they are confused. It goes against common sense. Shouldn't we know our bodies and report anything unusual? Of course, we should!

The debate is a medical one based on research and has to do with data that showed that teaching women to do breast self-exams did not "save lives," based on a randomized, controlled trial in Shanghai, China factories and a similar study in Russia. The Shanghai study tested whether breast self-examination (BSE) reduced breast cancer mortality. It was a 10-year study in which one group was randomly assigned to receive instruction and reinforcement in breast self-exam (BSE), and was compared with the control group who did not receive instruction. Detractors say that 40 percent were younger than 40 years old and the focus was on mortality, not early detection. Those who believe the study is important say that in the study there was no difference in breast cancer mortality, and BSE may have the downside of increasing unnecessary biopsies.

While the study was well designed, some very important issues limit applicability of the results from this study to women in the United States. Breast cancer remains an uncommon disease in China at this time, and doctors at the time of the Shanghai study had very limited experience in treating the disease. No mammography or ultrasound was available, and doctors had minimal training in surgical and medical care of breast cancer. As a result, the women who participated in the Shanghai study had health care that likely fell way below U.S. standards, and women could have died regardless of whether they performed BSE or not, just because they received inadequate treatment.

When breast cancer survivors hear the rationale that BSE doesn't save lives, they are most often outraged. How could a statistic of not "saving lives" be the basis for not recommending women know their bodies? While cancers diagnosed because of a lump will generally be larger than those seen on screening mammography, the risk of the cancer spreading increases the longer it goes without treatment. As such, it is important to follow up on any changes in your breasts as soon as possible, and "breast awareness" is recommended.

My non-scientific, personal experience has been almost universal in hearing survivors talk about the role breast self-exam played in their diagnosis. It certainly played a role in mine. That doesn't mean that breast self-exam saved my life or detected cancer on its own, but it motivated me to speak up in a variety of ways. Had I not been paying attention to my body and advocating for myself based on what I felt, I may not have found my cancer until it was too late.

Inflammatory Breast Cancer

An unusual, aggressive, and rare form of breast cancer, called *inflammatory breast cancer*, does not usually form a tumor or lump, but grows in nests or sheets. It may not be detected using mammography or ultrasound, so being alert to symptoms is important:

- Women with light colored skin may have persistent redness and discoloration that looks like a bruise.
- Women with dark colored skin may only have warmth or swelling of the affected breast without an identified reason for an infection.
- Thickening of the skin
- Dimpling or ridges of the skin, like an orange peel
- A rapid change of the appearance over days or weeks
- Retraction or turning inward of the nipple, or nipple discharge
- Marked enlargement of one breast
- A lump or thickening in or near the breast or under the arm

Swelling, warmth, and redness occur because the cancer cells block the lymph vessels in the skin. It can be misdiagnosed as a spider bite, allergic reaction, or mastitis (a breast infection which can have similar signs/symptoms, but fever is not usually a sign of cancer).

A doctor may recommend antibiotics initially, but if the symptoms do not completely resolve within a few weeks, a mammogram and ultrasound should be performed, and the woman should be referred to a surgeon for a biopsy.

#25: Pain is not usually a sign of breast cancer, but there are exceptions.

Though pain can sometimes indicate a problem (such as infection), and some cysts can be tender, pain is usually not a sign of cancer. Normal breast pain comes and goes, often with changes in the menstrual cycle. If you have pain in one spot in one breast (that you can point to with one fingertip) which persists over several months, it is appropriate to seek medical attention.

#26: Clinical breast exams (CBE) are an important part of an entire breast health plan.

A clinical breast exam is when a health care provider examines your breasts for lumps or anything else that might be suspicious. Health care providers are trained in doing breast exams, and they are an important part of an annual physical. Clinical breast examinations provide a 3 percent increase in cancer detection beyond that of mammography alone.

CBE is recommended at least every three years for women in their 20s and 30s, and then annually after that. It is important to note that your care provider is very interested in making sure they do not miss a mass or early cancer, but they examine you infrequently. If you detect a change, it is important to bring it to their attention.

#27: A facility that specializes in breast imaging will improve your chances of early detection.

Studies have shown that radiologists develop greater skill when they specialize in reading mammograms. A facility that specializes in breast imaging is more likely to have radiologists who have more experience reading mammograms.

Making sure that the radiologist has all the information needed to evaluate your mammogram and compare it to previous years could be the difference between early detection and delayed diagnosis. If you move or change facilities, make sure you take your films/images and records to the next facility and that the radiologist *has* them before reading your mammogram.

Choosing a facility that is accredited with the American College of Radiology will ensure that the physicians have met education and training standards, that the equipment is being maintained and checked for quality by a medical physicist, and that the technologists who do the imaging are certified. In Texas, Iowa, and Arkansas, facilities can obtain accreditation through the FDA-approved state accrediting agency.

The message of getting an annual mammogram has been repeated so often that we may become complacent or numb to it. I never fully understood the importance until it applied to my situation.

Even though I'd had a mammogram in my mid 30s, and went several years in a row after turning 40, I then skipped a few years. When I did go back, I went to a different facility. They did see something they wanted to watch, and they asked me to come back in six months. If I'd been going there regularly, it's possible they'd have caught it sooner.

#28: You should know your body and trust your instincts.

As important as any test is the vital power of a woman's intuition. We are born with this amazing gift, but we often learn to ignore it. We often sense when something is wrong, but choose to ignore it with rationalization, or put other's needs ahead of our own.

When our intuition *is* used, it can be life-saving. We've all heard stories of people who would not stop until they found answers, because they knew something was not "right." If you don't like the answers or lack of answers you get, keep searching. Don't assume that one test and one doctor could know everything. If you are concerned about an issue and are not satisfied with what you hear, let them know. They may refer you to someone or help you find the answers.

In my situation, there were times I used my intuition and times I didn't. When I felt that tiny pebble after the phone conversation with my doctor about my mammogram (they wanted to do a follow-up in six months to watch some calcifications), I was concerned enough to go back in within the week to see about it. When he didn't feel it and told me I could see a surgeon if *I* was concerned, but that he would just wait for the six-month follow-up, I stopped trusting my intuition. He didn't feel what I did and wasn't concerned. I questioned myself. Why would I be concerned? I wasn't likely to have breast cancer anyway. I was being overly cautious. Why would I want to see a surgeon? This doctor knew more than I did. This is where I stopped trusting myself.

Six months later, when I was in the dressing room after my follow-up mammogram, and the nurse told me I could go home, I trusted myself again and spoke up (see more of that story later in this chapter).

After being diagnosed, I trusted my intuition after seeing a wonderful, warm, and caring breast surgeon. I followed up with a second opinion at another institution. It was hard to do, feeling like I was hurting the first doctor, but for some reason I knew it would be important. With the second surgeon, an MRI was ordered and three more cancerous tumors were found. If I'd stayed with the first surgeon, perhaps I'd only have had a lumpectomy and the other cancers would have been missed (though, technically, the subsequent chemotherapy may have taken care of them). Trusting my intuition and getting a second opinion paid off in my situation. That being said, an MRI can overdiagnose cancers that would otherwise not ever come to medical attention and thereby prompt unnecessary surgeries and other treatments. It is important to discuss with your doctor if an MRI might be a good test for you for further evaluation once you have been diagnosed with breast cancer.

#29: It is critical to be informed.

It is critical to know your body, be knowledgeable about the screening tests and procedures you are asked to take part in, and why you are doing them. It could save your life.

When I went to that six-month follow-up mammogram, I was waiting in my gown after I'd been screened. The technologist came out and said, "You can go home now." I immediately spoke up and questioned her. "But I'm supposed to get a *diagnostic mammogram* today, and I have already paid for it." Her response? "Oh, we've already taken it off the bill." I pondered her words and thought carefully, not fully understanding the importance of my next statement, "But I have a lump." She questioned me, seeming to not really believe me, "Where?" I put my hand over the lump and she reached out to feel it, stating in a somewhat surprised manner, "Oh, just a minute." The next thing I knew, I was being taken back for a diagnostic ultrasound. The next day, I was diagnosed with breast cancer. Thank goodness I spoke up. Many told me they would have been relieved and gone home.

Knowing and understanding the difference between a *screening* mammogram and a *diagnostic* mammogram was a technicality I needed to understand. A diagnostic mammogram meant the radiologist would review my images while I was there and do more imaging if needed to look closely at the area of concern.

It was also critical for me to understand the limitations of mammography in my situation (having dense breast tissue). Understanding that meant that I knew further imaging might be necessary to clearly see a tumor. That is something I did not fully understand at the time, but thankfully, knew enough about to push for more imaging.

#30: There is a difference between a screening mammogram and a diagnostic mammogram.

A screening mammogram is one that looks at the entire breast using mammography in a woman with no signs or symptoms of breast cancer (i.e., it is a routine visit).

A diagnostic mammogram may include images of the entire breast, but the study is performed to look at an area of concern or because the woman has had breast cancer. A diagnostic mammogram should be reviewed by the radiologist at the time of your visit. Further imaging may be performed to see an area more closely, using special mammographic views or ultrasound.

If you have an area of concern, make sure that you tell your doctor. If you don't, further imaging will not likely be done. Don't assume that the tool being used is perfect and will find an area you were concerned about without you saying anything!

#31: Having dense breast tissue will lessen the sensitivity of mammography.

Film mammography sensitivity is only 30 to 55 percent for women with dense breasts, meaning that a film mammogram only detects breast cancer, if present, only 30 to 55 percent of the time. Digital mammography is more sensitive than film mammography at detecting breast cancer in women with dense breasts, but many cancers are still missed.

Results from the DMIST trial (a large study with nearly 50,000 women comparing film and digital mammography) found that digital mammography was significantly better in screening women who fit any of these three categories:

- Under age 50 (no matter density)
- Any age with heterogeneously (very dense) or extremely dense breasts
- Pre- or perimenopausal women of any age (defined as having last menstrual period within 12 months of mammogram)

No benefit was found for women who fit *all* the following categories:

- Over age 50
- Don't have dense breasts
- Postmenopausal

Many breast imaging facilities now have digital mammography, but if you have dense breasts, you *must* ask and make sure that you are getting a digital mammogram. Following is a story to illustrate why I say that.

After my diagnosis and treatment for breast cancer, I still needed to do annual mammograms for my other breast. I made my request for a diagnostic mammogram when I scheduled my appointment. I even mentioned it upon checking in on the day of the test, to the receptionist that, "I want[ed] to be sure to get a *digital* mammogram." When I walked into the examining room, I then asked, "Is this digital mammography equipment?" The answer, "No, our digital machine is being worked on." I replied that I would have to come back when one was available.

I was persistent in making sure that I was getting what I had requested at three different points. As it turned out, the machine was available in the next hour, but it was troubling that I had been very clear about what I wanted, but communication among the various staff or systems did not happen. This is an example of how important it is to advocate for yourself. Should I have had to be so persistent in getting quality care? No. But saving my life matters more. I do believe the more we all speak up and advocate, the better care we will receive collectively.

#32: Many women have dense breasts.

Over half of women younger than 50 and one-third of women older than 50 have dense breasts, a condition that lessens the sensitivity of mammography to detect breast cancer.

Breasts tend to become less dense as women get older, but some women continue to have dense breast tissue throughout their lives. Mammography is less sensitive for women who have a lot of dense breast tissue.

Dense breast tissue itself is also a risk factor for breast cancer, with the risk four- to six-fold higher in women in the extremely dense category compared to fatty breasts, and breast cancer is more likely to develop in denser areas of the breast.

Currently, mammography is the most common way to determine breast density. A breast self-exam or clinical exam cannot determine breast density. Though it is not perfect in determining exactly *how* dense the breasts are, the terms "heterogeneously dense" or "extremely dense" are used in mammography reports to indicate dense breasts. New techniques are being developed to provide more precise measures of breast density, which may more accurately assess *risk* for breast cancer. However, radiologists have been estimating breast density for years, and for most of us, the current measures tell us what we need to know.

Most mammography reports use the following terminology to categorize and describe breast density in one of four different categories:

1. Entirely fat
2. Scattered fibroglandular densities
3. Heterogeneously dense
4. Extremely dense

These are the BI-RADS classifications (American College of Radiology Breast Imaging Reporting and Data System) used as a part of the report. The latter two categories are considered dense.

Dense breasts contain more glandular and connective tissue. Less dense breasts are mainly made up of fatty tissue. Every woman has different amounts of the different types of tissue in her breasts. Breast cancer itself is made up of dense tissue, which means that on a mammogram, a tumor is harder to spot in dense tissue than in fatty tissue because the tumor looks a lot like the tissue around it. An analogy is often used to describe the way cancer looks in dense tissue on a mammogram: "It's like looking for a polar bear in a snowstorm," as both look white. Breast cancers are readily seen in fatty tissue with up to 98 percent sensitivity for film mammography.

#33: Ultrasound is an important tool in detecting breast cancer for women with dense breast tissue.

Ultrasound is used in the United States to evaluate breast lumps and masses seen on mammography. Ultrasound can also be used for screening in addition to mammography. Ultrasound provides an absolute increase in the number of cancers detected by 30 percent in women with dense breasts across clinical studies of over 50,000 women. Most of the cancers found only with ultrasound are small invasive cancers, and most are found before the cancer has spread to the lymph nodes.

For those at increased risk for breast cancer who are not recommended for MRI, ultrasound improves detection of breast cancer over mammography alone. MRI is more sensitive and better for those at high risk, but it is costly and insurance may not pay for it. Not all women can tolerate an MRI. Ultrasound is less costly, doesn't involve radiation, and may be easier for many women to tolerate.

A recent study showed that the combination of mammography and *screening* ultrasound, in women with dense breasts, has been shown to increase the accuracy of finding cancer to 91 percent compared to 78 percent for digital mammography alone according to the findings of the ACRIN 6666 trial results released in 2008.

This study used physicians, not technologists, to do the screening ultrasound. It was found to take an additional 20 minutes. At this point, most technologists are not trained to do whole breast screening ultrasound. It adds additional time to an already overloaded system with poor reimbursement.

> "Screening" ultrasound (looking at the whole breast) is not available at many centers at this time. In most breast imaging practices, you must have an identified area of concern that you, your doctor, or the radiologist has found in order for ultrasound to be used.

A limited supply of trained personnel and facilities offer *screening* ultrasound. Insurance reimbursement varies around the country, as well. However, if it is part of a *diagnostic* examination, ultrasound is nearly always covered by insurance.

If a woman wants to pay for a screening ultrasound, some centers may allow it, but most of the time it is not an option. Again, ultrasound is typically used to *diagnostically* evaluate areas of concern.

Researchers don't recommend that ultrasound replace mammography, but see it as a supplement, because some cancers are only seen on mammography. Mammograms are still important for women with dense breasts because they are good at showing calcifications, which are sometimes produced by early breast cancers. Ultrasound is not as good at detecting calcifications.

#34: If you have dense breasts, you need to be informed.

Back in 2004 when I was diagnosed, I started asking questions. I talked to the top radiologists in the country whose careers have been dedicated to breast imaging and the early detection of breast cancer. What I found was unsettling and motivated me to share what I had learned with other women. I soon developed a website dedicated to this information and had it reviewed for accuracy: www.KnowYourDensity.com. I started speaking to groups, made t-shirts, and spoke to anyone who would listen. My presentation was entitled: "When A Mammogram Is Not Enough." Being a pioneer in this area (speaking in public about breast density) was a lonely place to be, but women were enthralled; the medical community not so much. It was only after research came out, noting that breast density put women at higher risk, that my message became more acceptable. It wasn't enough that we, as women with dense breast tissue, weren't told that mammography had limitations and might not detect cancerous growths. Some still feel that we don't need to know because they are unsure what we would do with that information.

What we do with that information is advocate for ourselves. We can only do that if we understand our bodies and the limitations of mammography in our case. I remember talking to a major cancer organization about the lack of information around this aspect and how important it was, and the education director told me that they simply did not want to scare women. I'm not sure how knowing your breast density would scare someone, but what I do know is that knowledge is power—always has been and always will be. Knowledge may be scary sometimes, but it can save your life.

Knowing that you have dense breast tissue, and sharing that information with your doctor, may determine whether or not you receive further imaging based on your personal history.

In October 2009, Connecticut enacted the first law stating that every woman should be told whether she has dense breasts. Other states are following suit. Opinions in the health care field vary because they feel they don't have perfect technology to measure the levels of density. For years, they have been noting it in reports, estimating the density, but haven't shared it with women. They sometimes argue that women don't know what to do with that information.

The following is what that new law will require for women to receive in their report:

> "Your mammogram demonstrates that you have dense breast tissue, which could hide small abnormalities, and you might benefit from supplementary screening tests, which can include a breast ultrasound

screening or a breast MRI examination, or both, depending on your individual risk factors. A report of your mammography results, which contains information about your breast density, has been sent to your physician's office, and you should contact your physician if you have any questions or concerns about this report."

For myself, understanding the challenges of imaging with dense breasts have put me ahead of the game in working with my physician to detect breast cancer early, as illustrated in the stories in this chapter.

I remember arguing with a technologist years before my diagnosis that I wanted an ultrasound, because I had always had one in addition to my mammogram (I guess I had always had an area I wanted checked, without realizing it). I didn't really understand why, but knew that it was important because of my having dense breast tissue. She kept going back to the radiologist because of my persistence, and they kept asking me if I had a lump to examine. My reply was, "I don't know if I have a lump! That's why I want an ultrasound!!" They would not do an ultrasound unless I had a lump to examine. No matter how I protested, I couldn't even pay for one to be done. It's most likely, that if I had had a screening ultrasound those few years or even at my screening examination six months before my diagnosis, my cancer would have been found earlier than it was.

At the current time, here where I live (near two major comprehensive cancer centers), women with dense breasts and not otherwise at high risk, are still unable to get an ultrasound without saying that they have an area they are concerned about. I hope this will change in the near future, but it will take all of us advocating to make a change.

In Connecticut, law also requires that insurance pay for a *screening* ultrasound in women with dense breasts and in those women believed to be at increased risk because of a personal or family history of breast cancer.

The downside to this law is the shortage of personnel trained to perform *screening* ultrasound, and there are concerns about false positives. About one in 20 women screened with ultrasound may be recommended for a needle biopsy, and as few as one in 10 of those biopsies will show cancer. A false positive doesn't mean someone will be treated for breast cancer unnecessarily. It just means another procedure will be necessary to evaluate whether it is cancer—usually a needle biopsy.

#35: An MRI may be recommended if you are at high risk.

Women in the following categories are considered at high risk and are recommended for an annual MRI in addition to mammography:

- Women who are known or suspected of carrying a mutation in a BRCA gene.
- Women with a lifetime risk of breast cancer of at least 20 percent. This usually includes women whose mother and/or sisters were diagnosed before age 50, though many models are used to calculate risk.
- Women who have had radiation therapy to the chest after age 10 and before age 30, at least eight years earlier.

In women with some family history of breast cancer, a personal history of breast cancer or atypical biopsy, and/or dense breasts, there is "insufficient" evidence for or against screening with MRI.

As a breast cancer survivor, I get an annual breast MRI, which is highly sensitive to detecting breast cancers in women with dense breasts. Though sensitive, several negative aspects are likely to keep this technology from becoming standard protocol for the average woman. The rate of false positives is high, MRI is very expensive, and MRI involves intravenous injections of contrast while lying still for 30 to 60 minutes in a closed space.

Even if offered to women to be covered free of charge, I don't believe women would participate. Women have a hard enough time going in for a mammogram, let alone going in for an invasive procedure like a breast MRI. In a recent study, when women were offered an MRI free of charge, 42 percent declined. Women with pacemakers or certain metallic implants cannot have an MRI. It is reasonable to ask for screening ultrasound if you are at increased risk for breast cancer and have dense breasts, and are not eligible for or cannot tolerate an MRI.

#36: More sensitive technology will result in more false positives.

In using technology that discovers more cancers, there will always be more false positives, which simply means the results will be *benign*, or no cancer found, when biopsies are done on the areas thought to be suspicious. Most of the debates around imaging seem to center around this issue.

I have yet to meet a woman who would rather wait to find her cancer at a later stage than be subjected to a biopsy that might be benign (and the associated anxiety), but if you are a person who would, talk to your doctor about your concerns.

Another concern of policy makers is the economic burden and cost of these procedures to health care. However, a later stage diagnosis and the associated costs of treatment are some of the highest costs insurance companies incur today.

> My personal opinion is that any anxiety around having a biopsy or finding areas of concern that turn out to be nothing pales in comparison to a later stage diagnosis, lifelong, life-altering treatments, and early death.

#37: Many factors contribute to early detection.

- Be diligent with monthly breast self-exams, yearly mammography after age 40, and yearly clinical exams.
- *Do not* skip a year with your annual mammogram. Have prior exams sent to your current facility. Doing so will allow small changes to be seen. Detecting such changes is not possible if the previous examinations are not available.
- Go to a facility that specializes in breast imaging.
- Follow up any suspicious, palpable lump or other change in your breast with further imaging.
- See a breast surgeon* or surgeon specializing in this area to follow up on suspicious areas, when unsure.
- Trust your intuition.
- Go to a facility with digital mammography if you have dense breast tissue.
- Ask for whole breast ultrasound screening if your breasts are dense and if screening ultrasound is offered at your facility and they have the equipment and the expertise to do it.

I devised acronyms to help you remember to take action with SCRAM exams© and to be FEISTY© with your actions! Make breast cancer SCRAM and be FEISTY (i.e., determined)!

S Self-exam regularly
C Clinical exam by your doctor, yearly
R Regular
A Annual
M Mammograms—after 40, don't skip a year

If you have a lump, or other identified concern, be FEISTY© with your actions.

F Follow up and
E Evaluate
I Imaging (further imaging)
S Surgeon (with a breast surgeon when possible)
T Trust…
Y *Your* intuition!

---

*Breast surgeons are specialists in diagnosing diseases of the breast and are especially skilled in operating on the breast.

Chapter References

Berg W.A. (2009). Tailored supplemental screening for breast cancer: what now and what next? *AJR Am J Roentgenol*. Feb, 192, 390–399.

Berg, W.A., Blume, J.D., Cormack, J.B., et al (2008). Combined screening with ultrasound and mammography vs mammography alone in women at elevated risk of breast cancer. *JAMA*. May 14, 299, 2151–2163.

Berg W.A., Blume, J.D., Adams A.M., et al (2010). Reasons women at elevated risk of breast cancer refuse breast MR imaging screening: ACRIN 6666. *Radiology*. 254, 79–87.

Kopans, D.B. (2010). The 2009 US Preventive Services Task Force (USPSTF) guidelines are not supported by science: the scientific support for mammography screening. *Radiol Clin North Am*. Sept., 48, 843–857.

Pisano, E.D., Gatsonis, C., Hendrick, E., et al (2005). Diagnostic performance of digital versus film mammography for breast-cancer screening. *N Engl J Med*. Oct 27, 353, 1773–1783.

Saslow, D., Boetes, C., Burke, W., et al (2007). American cancer society guidelines for breast screening with MRI as an adjunct to mammography. *CA Cancer J Clin*. Mar/Apr, 57, 75–89.

3

When Someone Is Diagnosed

A Survivor Perspective on Being Diagnosed

Everyone's diagnosis and journey will be unique. People will have similarities, but just as we are unique as human beings, so will be our reaction to the diagnosis of breast cancer.

In sharing my reaction to the diagnosis, my hope is to put you in the shoes of a survivor. For just a moment, consider what that initial news would feel like in *your* life. Would it turn your world upside-down? Would it change the way you lived your life?

With each day, month, and year that has passed since that life-changing day of diagnosis, a new experience and perspective around cancer has found its way into my life. In fact, it's important to give a word of hope for those who are just being diagnosed, before they get to the end of the book. When all is said and done, you will likely find many gifts from the experience that will change your life forever. Among those may be a renewed appreciation for life; every day becoming a gift with less time for things that don't matter—and more time for what matters the most. However, many downsides accompany a diagnosis of cancer, and emotions of sadness and grief are a normal and healthy response. Taking one day at a time, one moment at a time, and finding gratitude amidst both the darkness and the light will see you through.

When the words came through the phone line at 8 a.m., I was in total shock, numb yet moving quickly and decisively seeing a surgeon before noon. I had a big conference to go to the next day, and I did not want to miss it. I remember saying repeatedly over the next few days and months, "I don't have time for this!"

I was on my way out the door to exercise, trying to get one more workout in before the American College of Sports Medicine (ACSM) conference, where other health and fitness professionals would be showing off their fit bodies. Being in the older crowd, relatively speaking, I wanted to be my best, and God only knows how important one more workout would have been to that end (tongue in cheek). So when the phone rang, I was a little annoyed but knew it must be important, and picked it up. The sound on the other end was chilling. The doctor was brief and to the point. "The radiologist called over here this morning. They think you have breast cancer and need to be seen by a surgeon right away. Do you have the number of a surgeon I can call to get you in?" Seriously? Not in my back pocket. And did he have any feelings at all here? I simply replied, "I don't, but I have a friend who was just diagnosed. I'll call her and call you back." I quickly dialed the number of my friend, Anna, who'd also been supporting our mutual friend who had passed away two years earlier, and who, herself, had also just been diagnosed (with breast cancer) a month earlier. Luckily, she answered, and we shared the irony of the moment. Our paths had crossed because of our friend Jean, and now we were facing the same disease that had ultimately led to her death. I quickly moved forward to securing a 10 a.m. appointment. "Well," I thought, "I guess I don't have time for a workout" as cancer began to work its way into my schedule.

That morning, my husband happened to still be home and had been watching in disbelief as I dialed numbers, one after another. When I got off the phone and said the words out loud in disbelief to him ("They think I have breast cancer!"), we hugged and broke down. I don't remember many times when my very macho husband cried, let alone sobbed, but the significance of this moment was not lost on me. This was a scary, surreal, yet sobering moment. We held each other for a long time, standing in the kitchen, shell-shocked, not wanting to move. But from that moment on, there was not much time for anything but action and survival.

I'm almost embarrassed to write about how hard the diagnosis was at the time because I'm very aware of what other bad circumstances many people are dealing with every day, much worse than mine. A few weeks after the diagnosis, I remember seeing a courageous burn victim, Jacqueline Saburido, on *The Oprah Winfrey Show*, who gave me perspective. She had been in a horrible accident, involving a drunk driver where she was trapped and burned leaving her without fingers, ears, a nose, hair, and much of her vision. If she could live her life with such grace and optimism, surely I could. And what I was facing seemed to pale in comparison.

However, as time set in and I realized what was ahead, the reality was overwhelming. I went back and forth between feeling overwhelmed and having enormous gratitude. The gratitude came from friends and family who were reaching out to support me. That was the greatest gift of cancer, to see the kindness and humanity shown at such a challenging time. It truly gets one through. However, what I was up against was difficult, and denying it was not helpful.

I had spent decades promoting good health and doing all the things I knew to reduce my risk of any type of disease. My real age at 46 was 34, and my cholesterol level was 140. I exercised almost daily, doing cardio and strength training, eating the recommended healthy, low-fat diet with fruits, vegetables, whole grains, and alcohol in moderation. I breast-fed both boys one year each, I avoided taking hormones or birth-control pills, smoking, or consuming caffeine. I managed stress doing the best I could to live a balanced life. Anything I had ever remotely heard might be associated with reducing disease was on my list. The rug was pulled out from under me in a sense because I believed, mistakenly, that disease could be prevented. Reduce risk, yes; prevent, no.

At the ACSM conference that first week, I was privileged to meet a Harvard physician who had just been through a year of breast cancer treatment and was giving a lecture to health and fitness professionals about what breast cancer patients experience. Because knowledge and information empowers me to make decisions, I welcomed it. However, learning the details of my impending treatment and side effects was difficult at best.

In addition to being diagnosed with a disease that was potentially life-threatening, I learned that I would most likely gain weight (and not lean body weight, but adipose or fat tissue), lose my hair, lose bone and muscle I'd worked so hard to build, lose muscle function/range of motion depending on the surgery, increase my risk for other health problems and other cancers, age 10 years in one, and possibly have anxiety/depression knock at my door. Oh, and I'd get to enter into the medical world in a big way, becoming sort of a "professional patient," as I call it. Needles, doctors, and hospitals—something I feared greatly and had devoted my life to avoiding! I don't know many women who would welcome losing hair, gaining weight, losing a breast, aging, and all the above, given the perceived importance of these things in our society. But of course, people kept telling me I was supposed to "be positive" (a comment and notion that is not particularly helpful and addressed in Chapter 8: Giving, Receiving, and Seeking Support).

Aside from physical loss was the loss of the momentum I had gained with building my business. It seemed to pale in comparison to the other things, yet it was a loss. We had built a beautiful home several years earlier that I had promised to help pay for, and this was a huge setback.

Mentally, learning that I had a life-threatening illness seemed unfathomable to this "healthy and fit" professional. I'd always imagined myself at 100 years old, dancing rings around the 20-year-olds. Though the prognosis for living 10 years was good, it wasn't 100 percent. If I followed the recommended treatment regimen, my 10-year prognosis was just under 80 percent. Sounds good to most, but for me, it challenged everything I'd come to believe and the way I lived my life. I was not supposed to have a disease at my age! Dying in a car wreck would make more sense than me having any odds of dying from cancer.

In my story I wrote for *Cary Magazine** the year I was diagnosed, I shared the way my less-than-80-percent 10-year prognosis and the treatment I was facing felt like:

*See the appendix for the entire story.

"We're going to line up 10 of you to jump off this very rocky cliff. We know it's scary, and you are scared of heights, but you have to do this in order to live. At least two of you are going to die, but not immediately. You'll all suffer quite a bit before that happens, but you won't know if you are the ones that are going to die. We don't know how long your life will be interrupted, but your mind and body will never be the same. Now, it's important to think positive. Don't get discouraged because the odds are in your favor. Get ready, JUMP!"

I felt alone at times, being afraid to admit how scared, sad, and overwhelmed I felt. I was supposed to be positive and strong, right? I had to still be mother, wife, daughter, and sister, holding everyone up, letting them know I was just fine. How could I expect anyone around me to fully understand what I was experiencing? The loss of good health in going through aggressive treatment, with multiple surgeries, including mastectomy, chemotherapy, and radiation over a one-year period was at the heart of my sadness. The first day of chemotherapy, I walked down a long corridor of very sick people. I cried, wondering how long it would be until I looked like them. It wasn't about them, it was about the values of good health that had been a part of my life for so long, and suddenly, this vision of health was crashing all around me. Thank God, I had some beautiful friends who let me grieve, and who supported me with understanding.

The imminent losses were hard to get my head around, but I knew I had to do one thing no matter what—and that was to survive. I had to survive for my boys and my husband. I had to survive to do the things I was put here on this earth to do. I was ready to do whatever it took.

#38: The period between initial diagnosis and treatment can be an overwhelming time.

It is hard to put yourself in someone else's shoes. Everyone's experience will be different because we are all different, but the reaction will probably depend on what type of cancer, what stage, and what type of treatment the individual is receiving.

Each phase of the cancer survivorship experience is unique and has its own challenges. The phase from initial diagnosis to beginning treatment is wrought with decisions, overwhelming information, and procedures in preparation *for* the treatment. This may mean meeting with multiple doctors—including breast surgeons, plastic surgeons, radiologists, oncologists, and radiation oncologists—to determine the best plan and course of treatment. Further imaging and/or possible biopsies, blood work, and other diagnostic procedures preparing for the necessary treatments can also take an enormous amount of time and energy. Combine this with entering into a world that is foreign to most with needle sticks, testing, waiting, waiting, and more waiting, financial and insurance issues, kind and unkind personnel, and a system that isn't always user-friendly. You can understand why someone going through this might be a bit stressed.

When I listened back to some of my thoughts on tape during this period, I was reminded of the cadre of emotions I experienced: exhaustion, depression, confusion, isolation (self-imposed), numbness, a sense of being overwhelmed, frustration, anger, gratitude, encouragement, hope, shock, love, disbelief, happiness, nostalgia, fear, and many more.

On the other hand, the level of distress will be relative to the diagnosis and the treatment that is being prescribed. Some early-stage breast cancers may only involve a lumpectomy and hormonal therapy, which is a blessing. Obviously, the more treatment and treatment decisions that have to be made, along with the corresponding time involved, the more a person's life will be disrupted and the greater the stress. No matter what the stage of cancer and treatment, a diagnosis of breast cancer will be a life-changing event.

#39: A patient navigator is a valuable partner to have throughout your journey.

A patient navigator is a valuable partner to have from diagnosis throughout the treatment phase and after. Given what you've read in this chapter so far, it's no wonder that patient navigation has become a vital part of cancer care. It is an area of service that is evolving and being refined each year. Some patient navigation programs use other survivors and volunteers, while others believe that only experienced oncology nurses can do the job.

Patient navigators can be found at local hospitals, large cancer centers, online, cancer support organizations specializing in navigation of varying types (usually non-profit), and as independent for-profit consultant services.

Depending on the type of service, a patient navigator's role varies according to how the organization has chosen to define a navigator. But the overarching goal is to provide support and help survivors know how to navigate or walk through the maze of what to do next, what questions to ask, find the right health care for their situation, and access the support network that fits their needs.

One of my favorite organizations is the Navigate Cancer Foundation (www. NavigateCancerFoundation.org), a national non-profit that works independently of any institution and can be accessed by phone or Internet. They are experienced, credentialed, and unbiased, helping survivors navigate through diagnosis, treatment, and survivorship. They are even there to support long-time survivors, family members, and friends.

#40: A diagnosis of breast cancer is not a death sentence.

A friend of mine told me that a colleague stopped talking to her after she was diagnosed because he thought she was going to be dead in a few months.

The majority of women diagnosed with breast cancer will live long productive lives. Eighty percent of women diagnosed with breast cancer have no signs of distant metastases where the cancer has spread beyond the breast and lymph nodes. Even women with cancer that has spread to other organs can live a long time. Treatments are available, and many more being developed, that enable them to manage the cancer like a chronic disease and live *with* cancer.

#41: Comparing breast cancer stories is difficult.

Because there are many different types of breast cancer, it may not be helpful to share Aunt Sally's story unless it is exactly the same. Knowing what type, what stage, and treatment they received *might* make the story meaningful or relevant, but people usually don't know that information.

When someone is first diagnosed, people often come out of the woodwork telling stories about people they know who had breast cancer and want to share. The stories often range from those living 30 years past a diagnosis (trying to give us hope) to ones where life was cut short (your situation is dire, and you need to take this seriously). About the only time these stories might be helpful is when the diagnosis is the same and gives a hopeful picture.

Understand that each individual case is unique and that comparing can be frustrating and even hurtful, particularly during such a fragile time. The story may also minimize the actual situation, which may be far worse than the comparison story, leaving the survivor feeling guilty that they aren't doing something they should.

#42: Breast cancer comes in many different types.

People think of breast cancer as being one disease, but there are different types. The only real similarity is that they all originate in the breast.

Breast cancers are typically divided into the areas where they originate: *ductal* or *lobular*. When cancer originates in the milk ducts, it is called *ductal carcinoma*. When it originates in the lobules of the breast, it is called *lobular carcinoma*. *Carcinoma* is a term that refers to cancer that originates in the epithelial layer of the skin or other tissues that cover internal organs, such as the breast.

Probably the most important distinction when getting a diagnosis of breast cancer is whether or not the breast cancer has spread outside of the area it originated. It is usually referred to as either *in situ* (self-contained) or *invasive* (infiltrating) cancer.

> In reading the rest of this chapter, you will see how many variables go into a diagnosis or prognosis of breast cancer. Each person's story will be unique, which is why comparing or sharing stories about breast cancer is difficult, because the comparison is not always apples to apples.

In-Situ Breast Cancers

DCIS or *ductal carcinoma in situ* is the most common type of non-invasive breast cancer. It means that the cancer (carcinoma) is contained (in situ) within the ducts of the breast. There is controversy as to whether this is a true cancer or more of a pre-cancerous condition, because it may not ever develop into a life-threatening disease. It does, however, increase the risk of developing an invasive cancer in the future.

LCIS or *lobular carcinoma in situ* is an area of abnormal cells that develop in the lobules where milk is produced in the breast. Even though the name has "carcinoma" describing it, it is not usually treated as a cancer, but as an indicator of higher risk that cancer could develop. It is treated as a "pre-cancerous" condition.

Invasive Breast Cancers

IDC or Invasive ductal carcinoma (cancer) means that cancer has gone outside the wall of the milk ducts. IDC is the most common type of invasive breast cancer and accounts for about 80 percent of all breast cancers. The term "invasive" is not the same thing as metastasis (see #46).

Other rare sub-types of invasive ductal carcinoma or IDC include:
- *Tubular:* Slow growing (low grade) and rarely spreads outside of the breast to become life-threatening
- *Medullary:* Common in women with the BRCA1 gene, slow growing and less likely to spread outside of the breast
- *Mucinous* or *colloid:* Develops in the mucosa of the breast tissue and is less likely to spread to the lymph nodes

ILC or *invasive lobular carcinoma* means that cancer has gone outside the wall of the lobules. ILC is the second-most common type of breast cancer, affecting 180,000 women each year in the United States, according to the American Cancer Society.

IBC or *inflammatory breast cancer* is in a category by itself, but is a rare and aggressive form of breast cancer. The signs and symptoms are listed in Chapter 2: Early Detection.

#43: The *receptor status* of the tumor will further determine the treatment options for the breast cancer.

A test will be done on each tumor to determine whether or not the cancer cells have extra receptors or characteristics on their surface that set them apart from normal cells. A pathology report from a sample of the tumor (taken at the time of core biopsy* or surgery) will determine what they call the characteristics or *receptor status* of the tumor.

Estrogen and progesterone receptor tests will show whether that type of cancer can respond to hormone stimulation. If it is found to be hormone sensitive, it has a better chance of responding to some of the drugs that block action of that hormone or suppress the body's production of that hormone. Following, these hormone receptor status test results are described:

- *ER+ (estrogen receptor positive)* means that the cancer reacts to the influence of estrogen in the body. The majority of breast cancers can be influenced by estrogen and often respond to estrogen-blocking drugs.
- *ER-* (estrogen receptor negative) means that the cancer does not react to the influence of estrogen in the body.
- *PR+* (progesterone receptor positive) means that the cancer reacts to the influence of progesterone in the body.
- *PR-* (progesterone receptor negative) means that the cancer does not react to the influence of progesterone in the body.

Anti-estrogen drugs are often used to block the signal for cancer cells to grow in hormone-sensitive breast cancers. These groups of drugs are called SERMs or selective estrogen receptor modulators (that block the ability of estrogen to "act" on the cancer cell, like tamoxifen) and aromatase inhibitors (that block the *production* of estrogen in postmenopausal women).

The type of estrogen-blocking drug used depends on whether someone is pre-menopausal or post-menopausal when diagnosed. Before menopause, the ovaries produce large quantities of estrogen. Drugs that block estrogen *production,* such as aromatase inhibitors (Arimidex®, Aromasin®, Femara®), are not able to overcome the production of estrogen by the ovaries, so they are only used in post-menopausal women. Even after menopause, women's adrenal glands and fat cells produce another hormone that is converted into estrogen by the body.

---

*Core biopsy is the removal of cells or tissues to examine under a microscope.

Each tumor is also tested for another receptor called *HER-2* or *HER-2/neu*. This abbreviation stands for *human epidermal growth factor receptor*. A special targeted antibody therapy (Herceptin®) can be used for this type of tumor.

Triple-negative means that all three receptors tested negative, meaning they would not respond to hormonal therapy or targeted therapy. About 20 percent of breast cancers are triple-negative. Even though there is not an additional treatment after chemotherapy as those noted previously, healthy lifestyle choices can be an additional weapon in a person's arsenal (see Chapter 6: Optimal Well-Being During Treatment and Chapter 7: Optimal Well-Being After Treatment). For more information, visit the Triple Negative Breast Cancer Foundation website at www.tnbcfoundation.org.

#44: The tumor grade is another piece of information used to determine the best treatment options.

Using the Bloom-Richardson scale as an assessment tool, a pathologist examines a sample of tissue from the tumor under a microscope and determines the grade of the tumor. Tumors that look most like normal breast tissue and cells have a low grade (I), and ones that are the most abnormal are given a higher grade (III). They look at three different features—tubule formation (resembling normal ducts), mitotic rate or rate of cell division, and nuclear size/uniformity—and score each one, which add up to a grade or score. The grades are as follows:

- *Grade I*: Slow growing, not aggressive
- *Grade II:* Semi-normal, growing moderately fast
- *Grade III:* Abnormal, fast growing, and aggressive

Grade I tumors have the best prognosis, and grade III tumors have the worst prognosis. Grade III tumors can double in one month, and are the most common tumors that will be found within a year after a normal mammogram because they grow so quickly. Other scales are also used to grade tumors, but the Bloom-Richardson is one example of a commonly used scale.

#45: Breast cancer has five stages.

When the pathology reports come back after surgery, the cancer is staged by its extent and its spread from the original tumor site. The stage is determined by the size of the largest invasive tumor present (if any) and whether cancer is present in lymph nodes nearby, or in other organs. Baseline scans may be ordered to complete staging. Determining the stage, along with other tumor characteristics as noted, helps doctors decide the best treatment options.

Stage 0—Non-Invasive Breast Cancer

Ductal carcinoma in situ (DCIS) is early cancer that has not spread outside the ducts of the breast and is *not* invasive or infiltrating surrounding tissue. Over time, most DCIS will become invasive, and it is often found together with invasive cancers. High grade DCIS will become invasive over a very short time period, whereas it may take a decade or more for low-grade DCIS to become invasive, if ever.

Debate and new research center around whether DCIS should sometimes be considered a precancerous condition (especially low-grade DCIS) and whether it will always develop into an invasive cancer. Every year, 54,010 women are diagnosed with DCIS. In new research conducted at the University of California at San Francisco, in 1,162 women who had lumpectomies and a DCIS diagnosis, researchers looked at certain biomarkers over an eight-year period. Only one in 10 cases was found to be associated with a future invasive cancer.

Stage I—Early Stage Invasive Breast Cancer

Invasive tumor is up to 2 centimeters (cm) in diameter and has not spread to surrounding lymph nodes.

Stage II

Stage II is divided into two categories, according to the size of the tumor and whether or not it has spread to the lymph nodes:

> Stages I-IV are "invasive," where the cells have spread outside the lobules or ducts to invade surrounding breast tissue. The sizing of tumors is only relevant for invasive breast cancers, not in-situ.

- Stage II A
    - ✓ Tumor is 2 cm or less and has spread to up to three axillary (underarm) lymph nodes.

        or

    - ✓ Tumor is between 2.1 cm and 5 cm and has not spread to axillary lymph nodes.

- Stage II B
  - ✓ Tumor is between 2.1 and 5 cm and has spread to up to three axillary (underarm) lymph nodes.

    or
  - ✓ Tumor is larger than 5 cm, but has not spread to the lymph nodes.

Stage III

Stage III is divided into three categories:

- Stage III A
  - ✓ Tumor is smaller than 5 cm and has spread to four to nine axillary (underarm) lymph nodes.

    or
  - ✓ Tumor is larger than 5 cm and has spread to up to nine axillary (underarm) lymph nodes.
- Stage III B
  - ✓ Tumor is any size and has spread to tissues near the breast, including the skin, chest wall, ribs, muscles, or lymph nodes in the chest wall or above the collarbone.
  - ✓ Inflammatory breast cancer starts at Stage IIIB.
- Stage III C
  - ✓ Tumor may be any size and spread to the chest wall or skin of the breast, collarbone, or axillary lymph nodes, as well as to lymph nodes near the collarbone or in the chest wall.

Stage IV—Metastatic Breast Cancer

Cancer has spread to other organs or tissues, such as the liver, lungs, brain, or skeletal system (bones).

#46: When cancer spreads outside of the breast, it is called metastatic disease.

When cancer spreads to other organs outside of the breast and axillary lymph nodes, it is either called distant metastasis or a recurrence, depending on when the spread occurs.

Metastasis is when the cancer has spread to distant organs and may be present when someone is first diagnosed or can occur at any time, even years after treatment has ended. After initial treatment has ended, and cancer is later found to have spread, it is called recurrent (or having a recurrence), meaning it has come back or spread. Sometimes, a breast cancer recurs in the same breast (referred to as a local recurrence), and that is *not* considered metastasis.

When cancer spreads or recurs in another organ, it typically means that a survivor will most likely be undergoing treatment for the rest of her life to manage the spread of cancer. The word "terminal" has been used because there is not a "cure" at this time. Most people who die of cancer usually die of metastatic disease. However, many will live with the cancer, almost like a chronic disease, for many years or even have times when no evidence of disease is present. Every situation and person is different. It can be a devastating diagnosis, but when the cancer can be managed, it can provide the impetus for some to live life more fully than ever before.

The most common places where breast cancer spreads are the bones, lungs, liver, and brain. Some of the symptoms for metastasis might include the following, but they are not inclusive and may not show any symptoms initially:
- *Bone*: Bone pain
- *Lung*: Shortness of breath or coughing
- *Liver*: Loss of appetite or weight loss
- *Brain*: Headache, blurry vision, or weakness

Other Important Distinctions

Breast cancer that spreads to the bones is not called bone cancer, but rather breast cancer in the bones. Lung metastasis would be breast cancer in the lungs, and so forth.

When breast cancer has spread to the axillary lymph nodes (under the arms), it is referred to as axillary node metastasis. This is *not* in the same category as systemic metastasis, distant metastasis, or metastatic breast cancer.

When breast cancer is found in the *other* breast, it is not a recurrence, but a new "primary" cancer that will require the same process of evaluation and treatment.

#47: The stage of cancer does not change from initial diagnosis.

The stage of cancer does not change from initial diagnosis, even if the cancer spreads or metastasizes. If first diagnosed with Stage IIA breast cancer and the cancer spreads to the bones years down the road, it is not called "Stage IV disease" but "Stage IIA with recurrence to the bones." I had always thought someone who had their disease spread, even years down the road, was called a Stage IV survivor, or that their cancer was then called "Stage IV disease." This is one of the most surprising facts I have learned in writing this book!

If the cancer has spread to distant organs at the time of diagnosis, it is Stage IV breast cancer. If a person is diagnosed at Stage IIA, and the cancer doesn't respond to treatment, and recurs in the bones, it is called Stage IIA with *metastasis* to the bones. Years down the road, it would be called Stage IIA with *recurrence* in the bones. However, all are commonly referred to as someone having *metastatic disease.*

The prognosis of someone with a recurrence would be different than someone who is diagnosed as Stage IV initially, which is why it is important to differentiate. No one can accurately predict how long any one person lives after a recurrence or with Stage IV disease, but it often means living *with* treatment for the remainder of life. It is often called a "terminal" state because a cure is not available, and it means that life will most likely be shortened. However, more and more it is possible to live for years with cancer as a chronic condition, managing recurrences with available treatments.

#48: Hormone receptor status may sometimes change with a recurrence.

A study presented at the American Society of Clinical Oncology in 2010 by researchers in Sweden showed that in nearly every third patient with breast cancer, the hormone receptor status changed during tumor progression. That means that the tumor characteristics of the original, or primary, tumor were different when it had metastasized. Based on their initial findings, testing of the hormone status of a new tumor might be important because treatments are chosen based on the characteristics of the tumor.

Aside from the hormone receptor status changing, you should ask for a new biopsy at the time of recurrence because it's possible it may not even be breast cancer. It could be a new cancer primary cancer, such as lung, colon, or liver cancer.

#49: Getting second opinions is wise.

Getting second opinions (or even third or fourth, if necessary) to be confident about your course of treatment is wise. Many factors need to be considered when being diagnosed with breast cancer. It is a complex process that requires meeting with a variety of experts. Opinions may vary as to the best path for you and your situation. Knowing the range of opinion before proceeding is important.

Even second opinions on pathology can be important. If you live near an educational institution that does a lot of research, taking your slides to be reevaluated is reasonable. Though extremely rare, mistakes can happen, and misdiagnosis can occur. I met one woman who had undergone an unnecessary mastectomy, in fact. That was probably a one-in-a-million occurrence, but it's important to understand that human beings can make mistakes. Human beings are the ones reading and looking under a microscope. Even when there is no question that it is breast cancer, the type of cancer is vitally important because it determines the type of treatment (hormone status of the tumor). If the cancer type is wrong, the treatment may not be effective.

> Unless a doctor informs you that it is urgent to proceed quickly because of the nature of your cancer, taking time to make life-changing decisions will ensure peace of mind and less chance of regret. That being said, common sense dictates moving forward as soon as possible, with decisions grounded in knowledge from your team of experts.

I know how scary it can be to go into this unknown world and seem like you are second-guessing the doctor. You may have a world-renowned doctor and cancer center treating you, but what I know for sure is that the world of cancer is evolving and changing all the time. Doctors aren't always able to keep up with every new procedure, test, and option available to you, especially if dealing with a recurrence or spread of cancer. I can't count the times I have heard someone say, "I wonder why my doctor didn't tell me about that (or ask, or check on that, etc.)?"

What I know for sure is that knowledge is power, and taking action on that knowledge can be life-saving. Asking questions and going outside the status quo can be very uncomfortable, but worth your life.

Chapter References

American Cancer Society. *Cancer Facts & Figures 2010*. Atlanta, Ga.: American Cancer Society.

American Cancer Society. A cancer's stage does not change. www.cancer.org/Treatment/UnderstandingYourDiagnosis/staging.

American Society of Clinical Oncology. (2010). ASCO Annual Meeting Proceedings (Post-Meeting Edition). *Journal of Clinical Oncology*, 28(18) suppl, June 20, 2010.

Singletary, S.E. & Connolly, J.L. (2006). Breast cancer staging: working with the sixth edition of the AJCC Cancer Staging Manual. *CA Cancer J Clin*. 56, 37–47.

4

Treatment for Breast Cancer

The journey through treatment and entering into the world of illness and disease was not easy for me. As I've said before, I had been fortunate to be extremely healthy my whole life. I did not take my health for granted and worked hard daily to maintain it. In fact, I was so passionate about my health that I spent a career helping *others* maintain their health and well-being (and still do). My oncologist commented to me once that he sometimes felt that it was harder for people like me to deal with breast cancer and its treatment because we had been so careful about our health. There is no doubt that the idea of putting needles and drugs into my body, feeling sick, or having multiple surgeries was about as far away from my reality as a person could get. It was a new world.

The good news is that I made it through and I am still here! Someone close to me refused all cancer treatment and her cancer progressed quickly, spreading throughout her body. She is not here. Although going through chemotherapy was not something I relished, it most likely saved my life, and I am grateful.

There were many gifts and lessons to be learned, in spite of the challenges. I have enormous gratitude for the experiences and people that touched my life during my treatment and those that have continued to touched my life because of cancer. However, I'm very aware and sensitive to how that sounds to women embarking on the journey. Gratitude? Please! Gifts? Don't make me nauseous! What I know for sure is that most women experience kindness from strangers that they've never felt before. Being aware of those acts of love and kindness go a long way in seeing you through your personal journey.

Into a New World

Soon after the phone call that changed my life, I entered into the beginnings of the treatment for my breast cancer. To be certain and to gather more information about the cancer, a core biopsy was scheduled. It was fairly benign and performed in the office, lying face down on a table (with an opening for my breasts) while they inserted an instrument into the only tumor they knew about at the time to gather tissue. A few weeks later, after a breast MRI showed a possibility of three other tumors, I was lying face up on a table as an ultrasound guided the radiologist to take samples from each one to make sure they were indeed malignant, or cancerous. Results were positive on all of them, so a lumpectomy was not an option for me.

After much discussion, we decided to do a sentinel node biopsy ahead of the mastectomy (often done at the time of mastectomy) because we wanted to see if the cancer had spread to the lymph nodes. This was to help us with the decision of reconstruction at the time of mastectomy. If cancer had spread to the nodes under my arms, I might need radiation, and would want to delay reconstruction until a later date.

A sentinel node biopsy was really the first major operation around cancer for me. Sounds like no big deal, but it's not like any other biopsy. Preparing for it required going in the day before and having needles injected underneath my nipple (ouch) with a radioactive tracer that would mix with fluids traveling to the lymph nodes. This was done because during surgery, the doctor would use a small Geiger counter to see which lymph nodes contained the radiation to help pinpoint the sentinel lymph node (where cancer might spread first). During surgery, a dye would be injected to give a visual marker as to where the sentinel node was. For me, this was a day surgery.

The period of time recovering from that simple procedure was more difficult than any of my surgeries, including mastectomy, oddly enough. Because it's considered minor surgery, the surgeons don't normally put in drains to relieve lymphatic fluid that builds up in the tissues. After a few times of having to go in and have fluid drained because of pain, drains were put in—something rarely done. I was thrilled to get them because of the excruciating pain that had stopped my life. I had tried to be tough, but I evidently had less body fat in that area, thinner skin, and lots of very active nerve fibers under my arms, which helped to put me into a very small percentage of women who have difficulty.

The night before the mastectomy was filled with emotion as I tried to have peace about what was to happen. Breastfeeding my children was one of the most beautiful gifts of motherhood I had experienced. Being able to calm, nurture, and give them life through my body was nothing short of miraculous. All the other obvious feelings about losing a breast were there, but not as much as this symbolic loss of a part of my motherhood.

I awoke to bandages and a lot of pain, in spite of a thoracic epidural block and morphine. I'm an odd bird in many ways, and when it comes to medical issues I'm that one percent of people that doesn't fit the mold or respond like everyone else. So it figures that morphine would not do anything for me, or that the nerve block wasn't very effective! And of course, no one seemed to believe me. I was one ornery lady.

However, when my surgeon walked in the next morning, I was sitting up on the edge of my bed, happy to see her and ready to go home. I wish I had a picture of her expression, which was one of surprise and shock at my energy and readiness to be moving around. I was ready to get over this and move on. Getting home, I did slow down a bit and experienced typical pain from such major surgery. I tried the narcotics, but again, they left me feeling worse than if I'd taken nothing, so I used over-the-counter pain medications. This time I had drains to collect fluid, and though it wasn't as painful as the sentinel node operation, the tubes to drain fluid were under my skin and felt like sticks had been implanted. Very uncomfortable. I was never happier as when they were removed. It was a hallelujah celebration. What can I say?

It is an understatement to say I gained a new appreciation for those living with chronic disease and/or pain. When I was going through a tough time over that year, I would think about the millions of people who live their entire lives managing pain or disease, and I would be grateful that this was (hopefully) temporary.

Chemotherapy began several weeks after my mastectomy. My close friend and college roommate, Robin, flew in from Texas to take me to the first day of treatment. What a blessing that was. Without her, I can't imagine how overwhelming the fear and anxiety would have been. It was the fear of needles, the fear of poisonous substances going into my body (even though I realized it was killing the cancer), and the fear of how my body would react. I had not yet learned to view the chemotherapy as a gift that would potentially save my life. It represented an assault on my otherwise good health.

We had a wonderful nurse, named Kim, who was kind and sensitive. She spoke to me like a child coming in for her first shot, which in a normal situation might feel condescending, but it was exactly what I needed. She was perfect. While I was being "infused" and entertained by this sweet nurse calling me sweetie pie, honey bunch, sugar dumplin', honey bear, and other southern names, Robin went to the hospital pharmacy and took care of other details to prepare me for the weeks ahead. She picked up my prescription for Neupogen® shots that I would have to learn to give myself. These would keep my white blood cell counts up (since they usually drop during this type of chemo) to fight infection.

So one of my greatest fears came to pass. I would not only become a pin cushion for others, I'd have to learn how to give myself injections in one of two places: my thigh or my stomach. Yikes! If only a film crew had been around to catch that. I'm not good at inflicting pain on anyone, let alone myself. It really wasn't painful—unless my husband tried to do it. Ha! Sometimes it would sting, and other times it wouldn't, so just the anticipation and not knowing if it would hurt would be a hilarious needle-inching-toward-the-skin-and-then-backing-away drama.

Soon after chemo began, I was told my hair would fall out. I had cut my shoulder-length hair to a short style a month earlier to prepare myself for losing it. I knew it was getting close, so rather than watch it fall out in clumps, I decided to take action and be in control. It was a private moment for me, unlike many who gather friends or family around to make a party of it. I took my son's electric shears and pretended I was Demi Moore, shaving for a movie role. If she could do it, I could, too, being the actress I am. After all, it would grow back. My son (18 at the time) reluctantly helped me with the final touches.

I wasn't one who liked going bald in public because it drew attention to the fact I was sick, my family didn't like to see me bald, and I didn't look good; yet, I would put on some outrageously bright colored scarves and hats, which were not always flattering. A certain confidence and power is required to be *au naturel*, and I admire anyone who can pull it off! I couldn't.

Losing eye lashes and eyebrows came later, and in many ways, it was much tougher for me. It not only made me look really sick, but the lack of them changed the way I looked. I'm a girly-girl, and eyelashes with a little mascara add that bit of femininity that set us apart from men. They are an important part of the female face in our culture, as are eyebrows that frame the eyes and face.

My treatment was on a dose-dense schedule, which meant every two weeks I would go in for my infusion (being hooked up to an IV). I did not have a "port" that some people have put in to help deliver the chemotherapy, which I was glad about. I've seen one too many people struggle with infections from them, and heaven knows there is enough to deal with! The day of infusion was long and exhausting. The trip was an hour to the center, waits were long (as it was a major cancer institution), and I had to see the doctor and have blood tests before I could begin the "infusion" of the chemotherapy. It was not unusual for it to be a 10- to 12-hour day. Friends and family that took me were invaluable support and company.

The day after treatment wasn't too bad, as I had steroids still in my system and could actually get a workout in. It was the third or fourth day, when the steroids wore off, that a touch of nausea and fatigue began. The fatigue during chemotherapy is unique and hard to describe. I remember describing it as the energizer bunny being wound up and winding down. I had a finite amount of energy that I would be able to use within a day, and it went very quickly. It wasn't like normal tiredness or fatigue that I could push through or rest and recover. It was either there or it wasn't, so I had to learn to manage it well. There were good days, as I would start to feel better around day 10. Planning and capitalizing on those days was important.

Side effects from the treatment, were numerous and often odd. One drug created deep itching in my hands and feet that couldn't be relieved by scratching, like an ant crawling in your ear. It would happen in episodes that came and went, but when they happened, I would pretty much lose my mind. We reported the side effect to the drug company, but they said they'd never heard of that particular effect. There were other times that I couldn't walk due to weakness/neuropathy in my legs, and I used a wheelchair (only at a few special events where I had to walk distance).

I tried to keep my routines as normal as possible, though there were good days and bad days when I couldn't do much. I even had speaking engagements during the height of treatment. I was determined to use my experience to educate and motivate women around breast cancer awareness, even though at times it was all I could do to get there. I even went on my first trip to New York City with business and got a personal tour from Margaret, my friend and colleague.

After chemotherapy, I scheduled the completion of my reconstruction surgery, which turned out to be a breeze, thank God. About a month later, I began radiation, after multiple consults with radiation oncologists. I was trying to avoid it, but based on my particular situation and cancer, a doctor said to me, "You need to see it as stacking the odds in your favor, Pam."

Looking back at this time during treatment, I recognize that I was in a "survival mode," and it was important to keep going and keep pushing myself. It was a time to reflect on many things, including my mortality and what mattered most to me.

I was interviewed on television during that time and had the experience of seeing myself on tape. I made myself nauseous with my cheery attitude. Why? Though it's important to be positive, the reality was that it was a very tough time. While I didn't want to be crying, being authentic about the challenge would have served me better. In general, though, I think the media, or our culture, wants us to be happy, positive survivors around the clock.

After formal treatment ends, treatment continues for some in many forms. For survivors who have hormone-positive cancers, the goal is to block or reduce hormonal influence with treatments of surgeries, or medications in pill or other forms. I had all three. The third, or "other drug," was goserelin shots that were given in my belly with a very large needle every few months to shut down my ovaries. I did these for a year or so before stopping. Then, after nearly four years of being put into menopause by the chemotherapy, I came out of it suddenly (and with a vengeance), so I ended up having a total hysterectomy to further block hormonal influences and deal with other related issues. As you can see, the journey continues well after formal treatment ends. I wrote an email to friends at the end of all of my formal treatment, which appears at the end of this chapter.

It is important to note that acceptable treatment and management of breast cancer is always shifting, as scientists and clinicians uncover new information that will impact better choices for treatment. Therefore, I made a decision to keep the discussion around treatment in as general terms as I could.

#50: Most breast cancer patients will have several types of treatments.

Most treatments include some form of surgery combined with additional treatments, which may include radiation therapy, chemotherapy, biological therapy, and/or hormone-blocking drugs. As mentioned in Chapter 3, all breast cancers are different with a variety of factors to consider when determining the best treatment plan. Most treatment plans will include surgery followed by one or more additional therapies.

#51: Different types of surgery are used to remove cancerous tissue.

Lumpectomy involves removing the cancerous tissue along with the normal tissue around it (until they find clear margins of no cancer). It is often followed by radiation therapy.

Mastectomy removes all breast tissue from the chest wall. Some women choose immediate reconstruction during surgery, some wait until they are finished with treatment, while others opt for no reconstruction. Radiation is sometimes done following a mastectomy, depending on the individual situation.

- *Simple or total mastectomy* involves removal of the entire breast.
- *Modified radical mastectomy* involves removal of the entire breast and lymph nodes under the arm.
- *Radical mastectomy* involves removing the breast, lymph nodes, and chest wall muscles. This type of mastectomy is rarely done.
- *Contralateral prophylactic mastectomy (CPM)* is a procedure in which women elect to have both breasts removed when cancer is found in one to reduce risk for developing a new cancer in the remaining breast. Little evidence suggests that CPM improves long-term breast cancer survival, though it nearly eliminates the risk of developing a cancer in the second breast.
- *Prophylactic mastectomy* is a procedure that is done when no evidence of disease is present, but it is undertaken to reduce cancer risk in one or both breasts. Women who have a strong family history of breast cancer, have one of the known genes for breast cancer, or are otherwise at high risk may choose to have their breasts removed.
- *A bi-lateral mastectomy* is a term used to describe both breasts being surgically removed.

Both lumpectomy and mastectomy may also involve the removal of lymph nodes from under the arm:

- *Axillary lymph node dissection* is a procedure in which between five and 30 nodes or so, are removed to see if cancer has spread to the lymph nodes
- *Sentinel node biopsy* is often done by removing specific lymph nodes under the arm to test for cancer, to reduce the need for a full axillary lymph node dissection. This procedure may be an option, depending on the individual's situation, when no evidence of cancer is present under the arm before surgery, and the surgeon is qualified and experienced in performing this technique. The first group of lymph nodes, where a cancer typically spreads, are identified with special techniques, removed, and tested. One of the reasons this technique was developed was to reduce a side effect from a full axillary dissection, called lymphedema, discussed in Chapter 5.

A full report with all the characteristics, including the stage of breast cancer, is not determined until the pathology or tissue samples have been tested after one or more of the surgeries described.

Before you make your decision about the type of surgery you will have with your team, it is imperative to consult with all the people who will possibly be treating you, as one treatment decision can impact another. You would want to meet with a breast surgeon, a plastic surgeon, a radiation oncologist, and oncologist. Understanding the big picture will help you make decisions that are right for you.

Issues Around Mastectomy

Emotional and Sexual Impact

For many women, this part of treatment is the most emotional and difficult part of breast cancer treatment. Even though they may have no doubts about having it done, a woman's breasts are unlike any other body part in what they represent. For those who breast-fed and nurtured their children for months or years, it is an ironic turn of events that an organ that sustained life could possibly take it away. The emphasis our culture places on the value of breasts makes losing them very difficult and can impact self-esteem, as well as a person's view of her sexuality.

I remember a story the first week I was diagnosed that gave me hope, from a fellow survivor who was years down the road. She shared that a young, single woman in her support group, who'd had a bilateral mastectomy with reconstruction, told stories of her promiscuity *after* surgery. She described this woman as vibrant and happy, saying the guys didn't care a bit, and it was no big deal. I am not promoting promiscuity, but the story of not being ashamed of her body and continuing to thrive was a welcomed story. With new reconstruction techniques, it is more than possible to continue life with *high* self-esteem and sexuality. It's how we view ourselves that matters. Working toward that end may take time, but it is worth striving for. Regardless of whether reconstruction is chosen, we are not our breasts, and our beauty and confidence shines from within. For those people who love us, it is a small consequence for still having us around.

Reconstruction may support a woman's image of herself and make a difference in her feelings around sexuality.

Reconstruction

A lot must be taken into consideration when it comes to reconstruction. Everyone's situation will be unique, but it is important to gather as much information, as early as possible, to fully understand the pros and cons of each procedure and how treatment may impact the outcome. Reconstruction can be done at the time of mastectomy or delayed until months or years later. Plastic surgeons who specialize in working with breast reconstruction should be a part of the team from the beginning. They work together with the breast surgeon, if done at the time of mastectomy. Sometimes, this can present a little delay due to scheduling, but in most instances does not present a problem and is well worth the wait. Women should know that being concerned about the appearance of their breasts or reconstruction outcome is normal and more than acceptable.

This area was important for me, and I eventually spoke with four plastic surgeons. After my first visit with a highly esteemed surgeon and his staff, I left and cried the rest of the day. Suffice it to say that bedside manners of the physician and their staff can make a big difference at such a fragile time. It's important to find someone with whom you feel comfortable working. The best in the world by some standards can be the worst in the world to a patient if a relatable human being is not behind the coat.

Mastectomy or Lumpectomy

Clinical trials have not shown a difference in mortality (how long you live) between removing the whole breast with mastectomy or lumpectomy with radiation. However some women strongly believe that their entire breast should be removed, regardless, and sometimes choose to remove the other breast even when the risk of recurrence is low. It is a highly personal decision for women and their doctors to make, if given the choice. In many situations, mastectomy is the only option, as it was in my case. I had four tumors in a small breast, so lumpectomy was not an option. I did not choose to remove my other breast, however. In discussing it with my doctor, I learned that cancer does not "return" or come back in the other breast, typically. It was possible for a "new primary" breast cancer to appear in the other breast, but I weighed the slightly elevated risk and chose to keep my breast. It was a decision I'm glad I made for many reasons, but I know many people who chose differently. At the end of the day, we must consider what works best for us by talking to our doctors and weighing the pros and cons. I encourage women to gather second and third opinions, if necessary, and take time to think it through.

#52: Three main types of systemic therapy are used in breast cancer treatment: chemotherapy, biologic therapy, and hormone therapy.

Systemic therapies are therapies that are either injected into a vein or given by mouth but travel through the bloodstream.

Chemotherapy

Drugs are normally given through an IV and delivered through the bloodstream to weaken and destroy cancer cells or stop them from dividing. The decision as to whether to use chemotherapy will depend on many factors, including the tumor size, grade, and the axillary lymph node status.

Timing of the chemotherapy is referred to as either:

- *Neoadjuvant chemotherapy:* Given before surgery to shrink larger tumors to make them possible to remove or to make it possible for less extensive surgery (lumpectomy versus mastectomy)
- *Adjuvant chemotherapy:* Given after surgery to kill cancer cells that may have gotten into the bloodstream from the original tumor

Biologic Therapy or Targeted Therapy

Biologic therapy, or targeted therapy, is a type of therapy that uses the body's immune or hormonal system to stop or slow the growth of cancer cells and keep cancer from spreading. Some are directed at specific parts of cancer cell growth and division, while others interfere with the tumor's ability to grow its own blood supply.

Those that focus on proteins that signal cancer cells to grow and divide uncontrollably, block the reception of growth signals, preventing more cell division and slowing the progress of cancer. It is usually combined with other chemotherapy, so is given intravenously.

Women who carry the HER-2 gene in their tumor cells, commonly use a biologic therapy called Herceptin as a first-line treatment (initial treatment of a disease) in addition to other chemotherapies. About a quarter of women diagnosed with breast cancer carry this gene.

Hormone Therapy

Estrogen promotes the growth of the most common type of breast cancers. For those who test positive for estrogen receptors (ER+), drugs are given by mouth after initial treatment to block the effects of estrogen on the growth of breast cancer cells or by blocking an enzyme responsible for producing small amounts of estrogen in postmenopausal women. The length of time on the medication varies, depending on a woman's individual situation, but can range from 5 to 10 years, with the type of drug used based on menopausal status (see #43 in Chapter 3 for more information regarding hormone receptor status).

In some cases, efforts are made to stop the production of estrogen by the ovaries via surgery to remove them or through drugs to suppress them and block production of hormones.

Hormone therapy may also be used as a treatment option when cancer has recurred or metastasized to other organs.

#53: Radiation therapy is used to reduce the risk of a recurrence.

Radiation is used to kill any stray cancer cells with high energy x-rays that might remain in the breast, chest wall, or axilla (underarm) after surgery, or occasionally to shrink the size of a tumor before surgery.

I love this quote by Marisa Weiss, with BreastCancer.org, who describes how radiation works on cancer cells and affects them more than normal cells:

> "Cancer cell growth is unwieldy and uncontrolled—these cells just don't have their act together like normal cells do. When normal cells are damaged by radiation, they are like a big city with a fire and police department and trained emergency squads to come and 'put out the fire.' Damaged cancer cells are more like a disorganized mob with a bucket."

Many emerging types of radiation therapy are less toxic, which give you yet another reason to meet with a radiation oncologist ahead of time to learn what's best for you in your overall treatment plan. Two general types of radiation are typically used. One is external-beam radiation therapy or radiation given from a machine outside the body, and the other is internal radiation therapy (brachytherapy), using implants where radiation is placed directly onto or near the cancer.

The length of treatment will depend on the method, but the way it is given will depend on the type, stage, and location of the tumor. External beam therapy is usually given over a period of five to seven weeks.

The preparation for radiation is fascinating. A mold is made of your body that you lie in, so it cradles and holds you* still during each treatment (different types of immobilization devices may be used).

They also tattoo small dots on the perimeter of the spot where the radiation beams go on the chest. It's done to make sure they hit the right marks each time to deliver radiation where it is supposed to go. It's also important to have a map for the future in the case of having to treat the other side or a need for radiation nearby so that radiation fields will not overlap the same tissue. In my case, they tattooed three little blue dots, one of which can be seen if someone looks closely, but no one has ever mentioned noticing them.

The great thing about radiation is that it does not take very long, and most cancer centers can accommodate busy schedules. A friend of mine scheduled her appointments early in the morning, so her day was not disrupted, and she was home by 8 a.m. each day. It's just a matter of changing into a gown, lying on a special table, and holding your breath or lying still while radiation is delivered in short segments of time. Once on the table, I believe it was around 15 to 20 minutes. It did not hurt in any way.

I received radiation after my surgeries and chemotherapy. As my hair started coming back in during this period, I felt like I was getting back to normal in some ways. However, for me, fatigue from the radiation and the cumulative effects of treatment hit me *after* the six weeks of radiation. Everyone reacts differently, but I often hear people who just completed radiation, comment that they hardly noticed anything other than a little fatigue. And then there are those that have a really hard time with their skin being very sensitive with burns. I did have a slight "sunburn" that was on the front of my body and went through my body to the back. It was startling to see a sharp geometric outline of redness on my back, since the radiation was given on the front, but it didn't hurt.

*As I re-read my words there, I had to comment on the irony of the words, "it cradles and holds you," which, I guess, could be used as a positive metaphor, as if tender or safe in some way, ensuring that I would be held carefully for just the cancer cells to be zapped away. I wish I could have used that positive image during my treatment! I believe my thoughts were fear of the damage it was doing to my body, instead of the cancer cells being zapped away. Positive visualization can really make a difference in the amount of anxiety a person feels.

#54: Adjuvant therapy is the term used to describe additional treatment after surgery.

Adjuvant therapy may include chemotherapy, radiation therapy, hormone therapy, or biological therapy, and it is done to further reduce risk of a recurrence, or cancer coming back. Sometimes treatment is used before surgery to reduce or shrink a tumor, and it is called neoadjuvant therapy.

#55: Nutritional supplements are not a treatment or cure for breast cancer.

Nutritional supplements have not been proven to treat or cure breast cancer. One of the saddest experiences I have had as a survivor is in watching women deny medical treatment because they believe they can cure cancer on their own.

Individual stories of women living a long time after having been diagnosed with cancer, and not having medical treatment other than surgery, may certainly be true. They may attest to how their natural treatments have saved their lives, avoiding the "medical" route with all its side effects. However, the problem, as noted in previous chapters, is that there are many different types of cancer that range from never likely to spread to those that are aggressive, spreading quickly to other organs. When a survival story is told, the person does not know the biology of the tumor of which they are speaking. Some early cancers are unlikely to ever develop into life-threatening cancers. But even non-invasive cancers can develop into invasive ones years later, as in this most important story that follows.

Several times during my treatment, I was approached by strangers, telling me passionately about a natural cure that I should consider. In checking them out, none of the "cures" had any randomized, controlled, human trials to back up the claims. Any research would usually turn out to be "in vitro" (in the lab) or with mice.

In addition, when the "cure" is applied to human beings, it may not be effective or may even cause harm, a frustrating aspect of research. I have found that when it comes to *natural* cures, there is almost always talk about a conspiracy of the government or pharmaceutical companies to not want the public to know about their cure, as well.

In fact our government *has* funded trials looking at alternative means of treating breast cancer. I am hopeful that one day we will have less aggressive treatments and/or cures for this disease. In the meantime, I am betting on medical science to save my life and discussing options that work for me. Some of the best medicines to work hand-in-hand with medical treatment for the best outcomes are exercise, managing weight, and eating healthy foods. However, they are not known to cure cancer by themselves at this time.

While I understand people not wanting to put things in their bodies and highly recommend making informed decisions based on each situation, I also understand that modern medicine is the reason we are living to an average age of nearly 80 years old. We live twice as long as we did in 1900 because of advances in medicine. According to the CDC, the top three killers then were tuberculosis, diarrhea, and pneumonia; now, they are heart disease and cancer. This is because we have "medicine" and advanced health care that saves lives. Is it perfect? No. I certainly believe we should not pop a pill for everything, but when it comes to infection or known disease that will shorten lives, modern medicine is miraculous.

I have been privileged to know many Stage IV cancer survivors of all types. They are living with cancer because of the stepping stones to treatment they are able to find. As one treatment is no longer effective, another comes around the corner that gives them more time. My close friend Suzanne has lived 12 years with colon cancer that spread to multiple organs, and she is living with cancer because the treatments have helped her manage it.

Because this topic is so charged with emotion on both sides, I want to share a true story about a woman and her husband who decided against recommended medical treatment that could have saved her life. It is just one example of many people who believe that cancer can be cured with natural medicine, vitamins, or supplements. I have changed the names and some of the less important details to protect identity, though this story is not unique.

> Rachel was first diagnosed with breast cancer and had a lumpectomy about 12 years ago. Chemotherapy or radiation was not recommended at the time because it was a very early stage cancer that was not believed to be aggressive.
>
> She and her husband believed that a previous biopsy had been responsible for cancer cells to spread and form that tumor. However, they believed that holistic healing, herbs, and vitamins would heal her and keep her healthy. Then six years later, she noticed some blood coming from her nipple. They decided not to go to a medical doctor, but continue on their healing regimens with their holistic doctor, and hit them harder. They were so intense that her skin turned orange from "juicing," because she had heard that the beta carotene in carrots would keep cancer away. After nearly a year, they decided to go to the doctor, because the condition was not improving. An invasive cancer was found, and the recommendation was for mastectomy and chemotherapy. They agreed to the mastectomy, but not the chemotherapy. Several years passed, but one day she noticed a lump on her neck. She was also coughing a lot. She went to a holistic doctor for treatment, but she was not improving. So after a few months, she went to a medical

doctor and found that the cancer had spread to her lungs and liver. Again, she refused treatment because they thought the chemo was too toxic and natural methods could cure her. They did not. Her cancer progressed, and her pain became almost unbearable. They went to a hospital emergency room and received medicine for the pain, but ultimately they believed that pharmaceuticals were bad and chose to keep fighting against them. She eventually ended up in hospice, where the nurses wanted to keep her comfortable with medication. Her family allowed this at first, but then said it changed her personality and they didn't want her to have it anymore. They felt like if she took drugs, it would be like giving up, and they still thought that there were natural methods that could cure her. They even went to another country to explore another natural cure (which failed).

Friends watched in anger and horror, helpless to help their friend. Even as she was dying, they were refusing any kind of medicine to keep her comfortable. Rachel went along with it, doing all she could to please her husband and family to the very end. She fought a painful battle.

If you or someone you love is thinking that natural cures will save their lives, please encourage them to reconsider and read this. Besides talking to an empathetic oncology professional, understanding the biology of cancer and all its varieties that require different treatments can be an eye-opening exercise. When it comes to risking what will or what won't save a person's life, it's important to know the facts and understand what oncology professionals have learned. Compare what evidence is available on all fronts. I would encourage people to get more than one opinion and use complementary methods (versus alternative methods) of healing to feel they are taking charge of their health (in addition to traditional treatment). The next few chapters will touch on some of these aspects.

#56: Treatment doesn't guarantee a cancer-free status or cure.

We have great treatment and therapies that *may* make breast cancer go away for a lifetime, but because there is no certainty, the word "cure" is not usually used because breast cancer *can* recur. Oncologists do not usually speak in terms of a "cure" because "cure" implies that the cancer will never return. In cases where cancer never returns in a lifetime, if the doctors could have seen the future, they could have said there was a cure.

Though every day of survivorship is a celebration, the "five-year mark" for breast cancer is not a home-free status as it is for some cancers. Half of all hormone-sensitive breast cancer recurrences occur after five years. That's why it is important to be diligent as survivors with regular check-ups and screenings. The highest risk is during the first few years; it then declines, but recurrences have been known to happen as far out as 20 years.

> The majority of women who are treated for early stage breast cancer will not have a recurrence, however.

According to the Society for Women's Health Research in their 2005 report "Science, Perceptions & Communication Surrounding Risk of Recurrence"*, most breast cancer survivors were unaware of their risk of recurrence.

In a meta-analysis (looking at the results of seven studies, in this case), women were at an appreciable risk of recurrence as far out as 12 years and for cancers that were initially considered low risk (not spread to lymph nodes).

For women with early stage hormone-positive cancer, they reported that one third would experience a recurrence, and half of those recurrences would be after the five-year mark.

*It is important to note that this report was in 2005, which may not be as accurate for the treatment regimes that are being used today.

In Summary Regarding Treatment

The following is a portion of a long email I sent to friends at the end of my treatment in 2005, which summarizes and gives an overall sense of what the experience was like for me.

Hello all!

It's me, Pam. I've been away for a while, "hunkering down" as my surgeon said I needed to do, for nearly a year, battling the treatment of breast cancer. I am almost 2 weeks past my last radiation treatment, and weaker than I've ever been. It's taken me by surprise, as I did pretty well during the radiation, but evidently the delayed effect lingers for up to 2 months... or longer... UGH! It's like having the flu, energy-wise. I thought I'd be getting my life back sooner, but I know, patience, patience. I will need to take more drugs to stop the presence of estrogen in my body, which fed my cancer, for up to 10 years. I am trying to give myself a break before starting them, as they have their own unpleasant side effects I hope to avoid (more weight gain, blood clots, other cancers, etc.).

I stopped with the updates after starting my chemotherapy, as the number of physical details became overwhelming. To try and detail the "state of affairs" was truly too much. Great days, good days, bad days, very bad days, and very, very bad painful days! I've been in a cocoon of sorts, really keeping the circle tight with just a few close friends and family. The energy required to just survive has been a learning experience, keeping me to really prioritize my activities on an hourly basis. I wrote my story for *Cary Magazine*, and as many of you know, they ended up putting me on the cover. That led to some wonderful opportunities to speak during the months of October and November, during the height of my chemotherapy, as well as a local ABC news story. Though it was very taxing to do, it was so worth the energy as I was able to meet many wonderful people and hear their stories as well. Because I work from home, I continued with some coaching and work for Wellcoaches®, which helped get me up in the morning. If you saw me out in the past year in a stylin' hat/scarf or wig, it was one of 3 or 4 places; Duke, an occasional movie/dinner, or one of a few business events I was passionate about that kept me living (or at those close friend's/family's houses—that ALSO kept me living).

I now am looking forward to widening the circle soon. My hair has grown to about 3/4 of an inch, my eyelashes and eyebrows are back in (YES!), and I was reminded by my mother the other day that I said

I would never complain about a bad hair day again...well, maybe not around her. :-) I am veggie soft and hope to get my physical strength back soon. I've had lots of setbacks due to treatment that have kept me from exercising as much as I had wanted... severe joint pain, neuropathy, and weakness to name a few…

[I go on to give a lecture about early detection and living strong, which I've covered in the book already.]

As for living stronger, I have to say that "Living Strong" for me at the moment means resting actively. A new term I've coined for myself. I remember thinking last week, how badly I wanted my energy and how weak I felt. I realized in that moment that the best thing I could do, instead of wishing for something that wasn't going to be (having unlimited energy), was to give my body rest and repair by being proactive and RESTING. I had to actually say the words (I am actively resting and healing my body!) as a mantra to get through the frustration and feel power to just lay down and rest.

Yes, living strong can mean many things. We not only need to stop in our busy lives and ask what is the best use of my time right now, but with our health; what is the best thing I can do for my health right now (spirit, mind, or body)?

[More talk about advocacy…]

Thank you for the love and concern you all have shown during this time. You will never know how much, even the smallest of gestures have meant to me.

Love to all and be well!

Pam

Chapter References

American Cancer Society. *Breast Cancer Facts & Figures, 2009–2010*, Atlanta, Ga.: American Cancer Society.

Chia, S., Speers, C.H., Bryce, C.J., Hayes, M.M., & Olivotto, I.A. (2004). Ten-year outcomes in a population-based cohort of node-negative, lymphatic and vascular invasion-negative early breast cancers without adjuvant systemic therapies. *J Clin Oncol.* 22: 1630–1637.

Fisher, B., Jeong, J-H., Bryant, J., et al (2004). Treatment of lymph-node-negative, estrogen receptor-positive breast cancer: long-term findings from National Surgical Adjuvant Breast and Bowel Project randomized clinical trials. *Lancet.* 364: 858–868.

Fisher, B., Anderson, S., Bryant, J., et al (2002). Twenty-year follow-up of a randomized trial comparing total mastectomy, lumpeomy, and lumpectomy plus irradiation for the treatment of invasive breast cancer. *N Engl J Med.* Oct 17. 347(16): 1233–1241.

Recht, A. (2009). Contralateral prophylactic mastectomy: caveat emptor. *J Clin Oncol.* March 20. 27: 1347-1349.

Society for Women's Health Research. (2005). Life After Early Breast Cancer: Science, Perceptions & Communication Surrounding Risk of Recurrence.

5

Side Effects You May Not Know About and What You Can Do About Them

Though patients are told about side effects in the informed consents they fill out before treatment, it is not common for a full discussion to take place unless questions are raised. There is almost never time for discussion around actions for preventing or minimizing side effects, even though the majority of survivors are at higher risk for many of these (weight gain, bone loss, lymphedema, and chemo brain). Of course, everyone will not experience every side effect listed, but it is important to have an awareness of each of them in order to monitor, prevent, or minimize the occurrence or impact should they occur. A few are so important to highlight, I felt they should have their own section.

#57: Weight gain is often a side effect of chemotherapy treatment for breast cancer survivors.

A most distressing side effect of chemotherapy is the one-two punch of weight gain. Nearly two thirds of women are likely to gain weight during treatment. The type of weight gain is the problem, because it usually consists of a gain in adipose, or fat tissue, and a loss of lean tissue or muscle—a condition called *sarcopenic obesity*. Even if the scale stays the same, the loss of muscle mass and increase in fat means that clothes may no longer fit.

Premenopausal women are at greater risk because they often go through immediate or premature menopause with treatment, which causes an even greater loss of lean tissue in a short period of time (and is said to age us 10 years in the span of a year). The average weight gain is between five to 14 pounds, though it can be much more.

Most people think of chemotherapy as a time of weight loss through nausea and low appetite, and though weight loss can happen, it is not the norm in breast cancer treatment. Researchers believe a combination of factors may contribute, from the steroids taken to control nausea to the energy balance between food intake and physical activity.

Steroids that help control nausea during treatment can cause the loss of lean tissue or muscle. This loss reduces the amount of calories a person burns every day. Steroids can also cause an increase in fatty tissue that is sometimes seen in the neck, face, or belly. The loss of lean tissue that burns calories at a higher rate than fat tissue, contributes to the weight gain.

Energy balance between food intake and physical activity may also play a role, because side effects such as pain, fatigue, and nausea can slow women down and make them less likely to be as active as normal. Regular eating patterns may change because of fatigue and nausea, sending women to eat whatever is palatable, and not necessarily healthy.

When you consider that 100 calories a day more than a body needs will equate to a weight gain of 10 pounds in one year, it's easy to see how weight gain occurs (one pound equals 3,500 calories). Eating an extra 100 calories a day or lessening activity by 100 calories can contribute to weight gain that slowly creeps up. And 100 calories on either side of the energy balance equation will not appear to be significant in your day. You can imagine how a 200 or 300 calories a day difference will add up significantly and quickly.

Being overweight increases risk for developing diabetes, heart disease, high blood pressure, and other types of cancer. In addition, *weight gain is associated with poor prognosis and increased risk for recurrence*, so it is important to make weight management an important part of the treatment plan.

What You Can Do

- Know that is it is possible to manage your weight and minimize a change in body composition (an increase in fat and loss of muscle) through treatment. Most women are unaware, so the first step is understanding what to do.

- Manage your calorie balance as much as possible through treatment and years after by following recommended guidelines for diet and exercise (in Chapter 6: Optimal Health and Well-Being During Treatment and Chapter 7: Optimal Health and Well-Being After Treatment).

- Strength or resistance training during treatment can help reduce the loss of lean body weight, or muscle, and keep your metabolism higher. The latest guidelines around strength training for breast cancer survivors have shown that it is not only safe, but important in maintaining lean body weight as well as offering numerous other benefits. Working with a physical therapist first, to learn about individual risk for lymphedema (see more in this chapter), wearing a possible sleeve during exercise, and getting baseline measurements of the affected arms are important safety measures to consider. Strength exercises can also be done at home using ones own body weight. Learn more in Chapter 6: Optimal Health and Well-Being During Treatment and Chapter 7: Optimal Health and Well-Being After Treatment.

- A healthy diet during treatment and after not only helps minimize weight gain, but can help the body fight infection and repair and build healthy tissue damaged during treatment. When prioritizing and filling the diet with fruits, vegetables, healthy proteins, and whole grains first, less desire remains for other less nutritious foods.

- Walking or other cardiovascular exercise for 30 to 60 minutes, five days a week can help reduce weight gain by burning extra calories that are necessary to maintain weight. Consider 5- to 10-minute increments throughout the day, if 30 minutes is not feasible. Always remember that some activity is always better than no activity.

- Daily activity plays a major role in calorie balance. One researcher from the Mayo Clinic, Dr. James Levine, talks about increasing "non-exercise activity themogenesis" or NEAT, which is all the other movement we do throughout the day that add up. Even fidgeting behaviors add to total calorie consumption. Dr. Levine has designed workstations that allow people to walk slowly on a treadmill and work on the computer. His work has shown that people lose a significant amount of weight over time by just increasing the amount of time during the day that they stand or walk slowly at these workstations.

When a majority of non-exercise hours in the day are spent sitting, it can be difficult to maintain a healthy weight. The difference in someone standing versus sitting most of the day can be substantial—between 150 and 350 calories or more per day for the average person. Following are a few examples of things you can do to move your body, if sitting is a major part of your day. Being conscious and aware of the amount of sitting you do during the day is the first step to making a change.

- Find ways to stand and reduce sitting time. Phone conversations are usually a good opportunity to move or pace.
- Take the stairs, when possible.
- Park farther away from destinations.
- Raise your computer so that you have to stand to work and alternate standing and sitting throughout the day.
- Wear a pedometer to track the amount of walking you do each day, including formal exercise, and work toward getting 10,000 steps each day. On many days during treatment, that number will not be possible, but after treatment, it is imperative.

#58: Breast cancer survivors are at risk for a condition known as lymphedema, which requires prompt attention.

Though not life-threatening, lymphedema can certainly be life-altering. It is an accumulation of lymphatic fluid in the tissues that causes swelling and pain when lymph nodes are removed and the lymph vessels are damaged or become blocked. It can develop as a result of surgery, radiation, infection, or trauma occurring soon after surgery or radiation. It can also develop months to years later due to scar tissue or other factors that block the flow of the lymphatic system.

For breast cancer survivors, living with this condition long term can impact everyday activities and self-esteem because swelling is typically in the arm and hand. It can often be managed with physical therapy, especially when caught early. For those who have to live with lymphedema, it may mean wearing a compression sleeve on a daily basis and going to regular treatments to manage the condition. When the swelling is irreversible, it can significantly impact confidence and self-esteem due to disfigurement and the limitations of joint movement and function. Prompt attention is critical if symptoms arise in order to manage the condition.

People at highest risk are those who have had a full axillary lymph node dissection, but even a sentinel node dissection, where a limited number of lymph nodes are removed, carries some risk. Other factors that put a survivor at risk are having had breast surgery, radiation, chemotherapy, and people who are obese or smoke, have diabetes, or have had previous surgery to the armpit.

What You Can Do

Be aware of early signs and symptoms, and call your health care provider right away to seek prompt treatment (request to see a certified lymphedema therapist).

Symptoms include:
- Swelling on the affected side in the arms, hands, fingers, or chest
- Skin tightness
- A sense of fullness or unusual sensation in the arm
- Jewelry that becomes tight, such as rings or bracelets

Prevention

- Exercise regularly with both cardiovascular and strength training activity. Gradually build duration and intensity of any activity or exercise, and monitor the arm(s) for any change in size, shape, tissue, texture, soreness, heaviness, or firmness. Listen to your body, and if you notice any changes, immediately seek assistance with a specially trained physical therapist. Seek out qualified fitness professionals, when possible, to guide your fitness program.
- Achieve and maintain a healthy weight.
- See a certified lymphedema therapist* in order to:
   ✓ Take baseline measurements.
   ✓ Learn about warning signs and preventative measures.
   ✓ Learn about special exercises to support lymphatic drainage.
   ✓ Discuss compression garments.
- Have blood pressure taken on the opposite arm (for bi-lateral mastectomy, blood pressure can be taken on the leg).
- Avoid trauma and injury to the skin to reduce the risk of infection on the affected side because infection increases lymphatic fluid (care with shaving, bug bites, sunburn, avoiding injections or blood draws, cutting cuticles, etc.).
- Consider compression garments during air travel.
- Avoid prolonged exposure to heat (hot tubs, sauna, long hot showers) or placing limb in water over 102 degrees.

*Certified lymphedema therapists are physical therapists who have had special training and certification around treating lymphedema. A list of these certified physical therapists can be found at www.lymphnet.com as well as more detailed information about lymphedema. Their hotline number is 1-800-541-3259.

#59: Bone loss is often accelerated and significant with certain treatments for breast cancer.

Chemotherapy, hormonal therapies, and other treatments for breast cancer can significantly accelerate bone loss, causing osteopenia or osteoporosis. Bone loss can be particularly significant if a woman goes through immediate menopause during chemotherapy, causing an even faster acceleration of bone loss than would normally occur.

For women who have hormone-positive breast cancer, part of the long-term treatment is to reduce estrogen that may fuel their breast cancer. The loss of estrogen in a woman's body during menopause can contribute to bone loss, so treatments that limit estrogen in the body add to this effect.

Personally, I lost 10 percent of my bone density and became osteopenic, which is a lower-than-normal bone density that many consider a precursor for osteoporosis. I did exercise during treatment, but I may not have consumed enough vitamin D or calcium in my diet, nor performed enough weight-bearing exercise.

What You Can Do

Minimize the loss of bone mass through healthy lifestyle changes:
- Make sure you meet your body's requirement of calcium each day and the vitamin D that will help you absorb it. Vitamin D and calcium supplements may be needed. Other bone-building nutrients include magnesium, potassium, and vitamin K. The best sources for these nutrients are fruits, vegetables, and low-fat dairy.
- Make strength training and weight-bearing exercises a part of your daily routine. Weight- or load-bearing exercise causes the muscles and tendons to pull on the bones, causing them to get stronger. Weight-bearing exercises include walking, running, walking stairs, or other sports that involve walking or running, like tennis. Strength training (minimum of two times a week for all body parts) exercises should fatigue a muscle within 10 to 12 repetitions to be effective. See more specific guidelines and information in Chapters 6 and 7.
- Avoid smoking, and be moderate with the use of alcohol if you drink (most recommendations call for generally no more than one drink per day).
- Discuss your bone health on a regular basis with your doctor. It is important to keep a close watch on bone density via regular scans, so if density levels fall, treatments can be begin to prevent further loss.
- Discuss possible medications with your doctor if lifestyle changes are not working to improve or maintain your bone health. A group of drugs called biphosphonates have been approved by the U.S. Food and Drug Administration to treat osteoporosis and are often recommended. Other types of medications are being studied to protect bones during and after treatment.

#60: Standard chemotherapies and radiation can cause cardiotoxicity, which can occur during treatment or decades later.

Though it has been known for decades that certain therapies can cause damage to the heart, focus has increased around cardiac toxicities for breast cancer survivors and how they may contribute to cardiovascular disease that may not show up until years down the road. Though it is not a common occurrence, it is vital for physicians and survivors to be aware of the risk and monitor cardiovascular health.

Chemotherapies most often associated with breast cancer treatment are the anthracycline doxorubicin (trade name Adriamycin®), trastuzumab (Herceptin®), and sometimes high dose cyclophosphamide (Cytoxan®) that can cause cardiomyopathy (weakening of the heart muscle), or left ventricle dysfunction or heart failure. Irregular heartbeats or arrhythmias have been associated with paclitaxel (Taxol®). In a study by Doyle, et al. women 65 years and older who had chemotherapy had a 10 percent overall risk of cardiomyopathy at five years out compared to a control group at 4 percent for women the same age who had not had chemotherapy.

- Doses vary by individual, so it is important to keep a record of your treatment doses. The higher the doses given over time, the higher the risk, though even low amounts can result in problems.
- For anthracyclines, doses greater than 550mg/m2 are associated with more risk, but doses as low as 250mg/m2 have resulted in changes. Most initial protocols keep doses in the lower range.
- Changes can be detected on tests like an ECHO or MUGA (multi-gated acquisition scan, or radionuclide angiography) scans, but newer, more sensitive technologies are on the horizon
- Problems can sometimes be subclinical (not showing significant symptoms) and not become an issue for years

Radiation to the left chest wall can increase risk for heart damage, but current protocols are very careful to minimize exposure to the heart, so it is unlikely to happen. However, women who have preexisting heart disease and have also received Adriamycin or Cytoxan may have an additive or synergistic effect.

Radiation can also impact the lungs and cause scarring (fibrosis) or inflammation (pheumonitis). Evaluations that might be considered: chest x-ray, CAT scans of the chest, or pulmonary function tests.

Patients with any of the following characteristics are considered to be at elevated risk for developing cardiac complications from their cancer therapy:

- Having been treated with the anthracyclines doxorubicin > 300 mg/m2, epirubicin > 600 mg/m2, mitoxantrone > 100 mg/m2, or combined mediastinal radiation and anthracyclines
- Having a tumor close to the heart
- Having radiation treatment prior to 1970
- Receiving total radiation > 35 Gy (Gray is the unit measure of absorbed radiation)
- Having a daily dose of radiation fraction > 2 Gy/day
- Being younger than 18 or older than 65 years of age at the time of treatment
- Having preexisting cardiac risk factors (hypertension or coronary artery disease)
- Being pregnant or contemplating pregnancy after therapy with any anthracycline or mediastinal irradiation
- Living more than 10 years since completing therapy

What You Can Do

- Keep a list of the therapies and doses you received during treatment so you can share them with your primary physician, or others as needed.
- If you will receive any dose of anthracyclines, have a baseline ECHO or MUGA scan before treatment begins that will look at left ventricular function. Periodic follow-up evaluation is recommended throughout treatment, and then at five-year intervals if no changes are seen. If subtle changes are seen, a referral to a specialist or more frequent monitoring is recommended.
- Report any of the following symptoms to your doctor:
  ✓ Shortness of breath (with or without exertion)
  ✓ Chest heaviness
  ✓ Chest pain
  ✓ Rapid heart beat or palpitations
  ✓ Dizziness/lightheadedness
  ✓ Swelling of the arms or legs
  ✓ Fatigue
  ✓ Difficulty breathing when lying down
- Make healthy lifestyle choices that will keep your cardiovascular system strong, such as exercising regularly, eating healthy foods, maintaining a healthy weight, and avoiding smoking and drug use.
- Researchers believe that exercise during treatment may have a protective effect on the heart and is under investigation.

#61: Chemobrain is real.

Women going through chemotherapy will often experience significant cognitive changes that are commonly referred to as "chemo brain" or "chemo fog." For the overwhelming majority, this is a short-term and fully reversible side effect.

Though survivors talk about chemo brain regularly, it is a major side effect that is not often discussed or addressed with medical providers, though that is changing. Research is now showing that a significant number of women experience both short- and long-term changes after chemotherapy that can sometimes last for years. New research in other cancer types has shown that chemo brain lasted five years or longer, and they believe it will apply to breast cancer survivors as well. It is now a hot area of research, not only to determine its prevalence, but also to learn what might minimize its impact.

Scientists are not sure of the exact cause, but hypothesize it may be a combination of factors. The physiological impact of some common side effects such as sudden onset of menopause (if pre-menopausal), disrupted sleep patterns, estrogen deficiency, fatigue, anxiety, depression, and other lifestyle habits like sedentary behavior, or poor diet may all contribute and play a synergistic role.

In *Your Brain After Chemo: A Practical Guide to Lifting the Fog and Getting Back Your Focus*, Dan Silverman and Idelle Davidson describe in great detail the cognitive domains or areas that may be impacted:

- *Executive functioning:* Planning ahead, solving problems, making decisions, multitasking, retrieving information, interpreting events and reacting appropriately
- *Information processing speed:* Taking longer to learn new things, responding or reacting (which can also impact word finding)
- *Language:* Word retrieval or word finding, speed and fluency of language
- *Attention:* Difficulty with attention and concentration
- *Memory:* Losing keys, remembering names, where you parked

The book is a treasure chest that explains the hows and whys behind these challenges in great detail and offers practical strategies to improve memory and focus. More than anything, it offers the questions a person might ask her oncologist about her particular treatment regimen and how it might impact cognitive functioning.

What You Can Do

Before Chemotherapy

- Talk to your doctor about what impact the treatment program you will be on may have on your cognitive functioning, and weigh it against your own personal risk.

- Discuss the possibility of baseline testing before chemotherapy and at various intervals during and after treatment (see *Your Brain After Chemo* for questions to ask your doctor).

During and After Chemotherapy

- Do all you can to incorporate healthy lifestyle habits within your routines, as discussed throughout this book:
  - ✓ Exercise.
  - ✓ Eat a healthy diet with colorful fruits and vegetables.
  - ✓ Get enough sleep.
  - ✓ Manage stress.
- Challenge and exercise your brain with puzzles, memory exercises, learning new information, or other stimulating tasks.
- Have routines, and pick certain places to leave common items like keys. I always have my keys in one place in my purse. They stay there unless they are in the ignition!
- Use a personal calendar or planner on which all activities and phone numbers are kept, and check it daily. Personally, I check my calendar frequently throughout the day to remember client appointments and meeting times.
- Keep a log of phone conversations with notes for work and personal life. Keep them in one pocket journal so that everything is in one place.
- Meet with a neurologist, psycho-neurologist, or psychologist to evaluate and suggest ways to manage the changes.
- Keep up to date with the latest research and clinical trials that may be available, as this is a fairly new area of research. Scientists are looking into ways to protect the brain during chemotherapy as well as ways to help survivors improve deficits that may have developed.
- Let others around you know about this side effect that you are learning to manage. Having "chemo brain" doesn't mean you are less intelligent, but it may mean you are not yourself for a while. Telling people may lessen the stress and anxiety of recalling information or words or trying to find your keys, if those around you understand.

Personally, when I speak about this side effect, people laugh and say that they experience the same thing, and that it is just about getting older. While that may be true to some extent, it is a sudden change that is on a scale of greater severity. The impact may be more intense by those who have to use their verbal and cognitive skills professionally.

When I think back of the time during and after treatment, I kept saying I was not myself. I could not put my finger on it, and I wanted people to understand that this was not the person I had always been (especially those with whom I had just met). I don't know how people perceived those words, but it made me feel better.

I look back on some of the decisions, statements, and other actions I made during this time, and I am quite embarrassed. I know that I am a strong, capable, intelligent woman, but I'm aware that others may have seen sides of me that made them wonder. Between my word-finding challenges and putting my thoughts into words in a way that were articulate, I know I sometimes appeared less than capable. I am still challenged by these things, but not to the extent I felt them early in my treatment. Yes, I have written a book, but it has been one of the most challenging, yet rewarding things I have ever done!

Some of the stories I've heard from survivors who have experienced significant cognitive changes are heartbreaking. The impact of this side effect can affect jobs and careers, not to mention self-esteem and confidence. If you or someone you love has experienced problems in this area, I urge you to seek help earlier rather than later (with a neurologist, psychologist, or psycho-neurologist, or other medical provider), and most of all, have compassion for yourself and those dealing with this issue.

Chapter References

American Cancer Society. Breast cancer chemo changes body composition. Atlanta, Ga.: American Cancer Society.

American Society of Clinical Oncology (ASCO) www.cancer.net

Blaes, A.H. (2010). Cardiac complications from cancer therapy. *Minnesota Medicine.* October.

Demark-Wahnefried, W., Peterson, B.L., Winer, E.P., et al (2001). Changes in weight, body composition, and factors influencing energy balance among premenopausal breast cancer patients receiving adjuvant chemotherapy. *J Clin Oncol.* 19: 2381–2389.

Doyle, J.J., Neugut, A.I., Jacobson, J.S., Grann, V.R., & Hershman, D.L. (2005). Chemotherapy and cardiotoxicity in older breast cancer patients: a population-based study. *J Clin Oncol.* 23: 8597–8605.

Hewitt, M., Greenfield, S., Stovall, E. [Eds.]. (2006). *From Cancer Patient to Cancer Survivor: Lost in Transition.* Washington, D.C.: National Academies Press.

Horning, S. & Rosenbaum, E.H. (2009). Symptomatic problems in cancer survivors. Aug. 23. Retrieved on August 12, 2011 from www.cancersupportivecare.com/Survivorship/symptom.html.

Levine, J.A., Schleusner, S.J., Jensen, M.D. (2000). Energy expenditure of non-exercise activity. *Am J Clin Nutr.* 72: 1451–1454.

LIVE**STRONG** Care Plan powered by Penn Medicine's OncoLink www.LivestrongCarePlan.org.

The www.lymphnet.org National Lymphedema Network.

Panjari, M., Bell, R.J., & Davis, S.R. (2011). Sexual function after breast cancer. *J Sex Med.* 8: 294–302.

Rosenbaum, E.H. (2008). Cancer treatment side effects and solutions. August 2. Retrieved on August 12, 2011 from www.cancersupportivecare.com/Survivor/comorbid.html.

Segal, R., Evans, W., Johnson, D., et al (2001). Structured exercise improves physical functioning in women with stages I and II breast cancer: Results of a randomized controlled trial. *J Clin Oncol.* 19: 657–665.

Syrjala, K.L., Artherholt, S.B., Kurland, B.F., Langer, S.L., Roth-Roemer, S., Elrod, J.B., & Dikmen, S. (2011). Prospective neurocognitive function over 5 years after allogeneic hematopoietic cell transplantation for cancer survivors compared with matched controls at 5 years, *J Clin Oncol.* June 10:29 (17): 2397-404.

Wefel, J.S., Saleeba, A.K., Buzdar, A.U., & Meyers, C.A. (2010). Acute and late onset cognitive dysfunction associated with chemotherapy in women with breast cancer. *Cancer,* 116: 3348–3356. doi: 10.1002/cncr.25098.

6

Optimal Well-Being During Treatment

It may sound like an oxymoron to talk about "well-being" during chemotherapy or other treatment, but doing what you can to *optimize* well-being, given the circumstance, fosters hopeful thoughts, feelings, and actions. The definition of well-being is "the state of being comfortable, healthy, or happy" and we can do a lot as survivors to impact all of those areas.

Some of the hardest sections to write and condense have been the chapters on optimal well-being (Chapters 6 and 7) because they are my areas of focus in my practice as a wellness coach, fitness professional, and speaker. The subject deserves its own book, but for now, I've taken the best of what I've learned from the volumes of information, experts, and personal experiences that I believe will help survivors the most. What will follow is in addition to the information on side effects in Chapter 5: Side Effects You May Not Know About and What You Can Do About Them and the vital steps needed to ensure well-being.

Being at the American College of Sports Medicine conference the week of my diagnosis, I was able to attend a session designed for fitness professionals to learn about breast cancer, its treatments, and the impact on the body. As mentioned earlier, the session was led by a Harvard breast surgeon and survivor, who had just completed a year of treatment. She knew intimately what was important for professionals to hear.

It was overwhelming to learn how my body would be broken down in order to treat this horrible disease. Seeing it in writing, here, may also be difficult for some. While it *is* difficult, knowledge is power. Having knowledge ahead of time and learning what you can do to possibly minimize or reduce problems is imperative.

The information I learned at the conference piqued my curiosity and I sought to learn more by speaking to top researchers around the country. One in particular left a lasting impression. When reflecting the recommendations she'd just given me ("So I should do strength training when I feel like it?"), she responded that no, I needed to do it whether I felt like it or not. I was taken aback. I had always been proactive with my health, but the role I would need to play was far greater than anything I'd imagined.

Sitting back and letting nature (or medicine) takes its course would have major consequences. There was much I needed to do that no doctor or drug could do for me. Further, my oncology team was not telling me these types of things.

Hope is having some control over your circumstances. Taking charge of your well-being is the ultimate example of fostering hope. With a pathway to follow, it essentially gives us hope that our lives, our situation, and/or our health can be improved. It energizes us!

Please understand that nothing here is about a hard-and-fast rule. Each of us has our own way of being in the world. Take what science and experiences have taught us, use what works for you, and leave the rest. Chapters 6 and 7 are learning about what *you* can do to minimize challenges and optimize well-being.

#62: You will get your life back, so for the meantime, hunker down, fight this disease, and take care of yourself.

It may be surprising to hear me start with this, but the key message is one that will help with your overall well-being: *patience*. A physician told me this, in a loving way, letting me know that it would not necessarily be an easy path, but one I could manage if I understood things might be different for a while. When undergoing this upheaval of treatment in your life, you will have times when it seems like the world is going on without you and life is passing you by. Be patient, and know that this time will pass and you will have your life back once again. It's not to suggest that you can't live life and experience wonderful things during this time, because you will. Again, everyone is individual in their experience, but it may mean that fatigue or other side effects may sideline you here and there. Just the time alone, managing doctor appointments and treatments, is a major disruption. Accepting that life will be disrupted for a bit, while learning to take care of yourself, and focusing on what is good and right in your life, will help tremendously.

A coach and good friend of mine, named Susan, had extensive surgery for a third cancer (none of them breast) and spoke to this in her blog:

> "Life seemed to come to a screeching halt for a while. I got off the merry-go-round that we all seem to be on and thought my world was going to fall apart. But then, lo and behold, after it was all over with, I managed to get right back on the merry-go-round, almost as if nothing had happened! I saw that my world was intact, nothing much had changed, and most of the things that I put on hold were just waiting for me to pick up where I left off. It is so amazing. Life went on for everyone else; it was just temporarily on hold for me."

Susan is a very positive person who has been through much, and is an inspiration. She has lived with lymphedema as a result of prior cancer treatments, wearing a compression sleeve on her leg most of her life. She exercises and swims regularly and is the perfect example of good health. When she says she got back to her life "almost as if nothing had happened," she would be the first to tell you that cancer can have a huge impact on your life and change it, but getting back to the world, the routine of life, and opportunities will be waiting.

So life may be a bit different for a while, but choosing a mindset of "this too will pass" and that you are hunkering down for a bit to take care of yourself can help with patience. This time can be an opportunity for taking advantage of every possible nurturing thought, action, or supportive service available to improve optimal health and well-being habits that may well last the rest of your life.

#63: Managing side effects helps you stick with lifesaving treatments and be comfortable.

Staying connected with your health care team about side effects from treatment could make the difference between misery and comfort, life and death. As many as 40 percent of patients will quit treatment because of poor side effect management.

One of the most heartbreaking things I've witnessed is when survivors are suffering needlessly, unaware that there are ways to manage the symptoms they are dealing with. Communicating with the health care provider clearly, honestly, and without delay can make the difference in a manageable experience and one that is extremely difficult. Time spent on unnecessary pain, stress, and discomfort can prevent more important daily tasks (work, daily activities, etc.) and self-care to take place (exercise, sleep, other support services and activities, etc.).

Providers may not always remember to tell you what numbers to call should you have a question or problem. There may be a triage nurse or a nurse line you can call in between treatments. Sometimes, just hearing that what you are experiencing is normal can be reassuring and put your mind at ease.

All treatments will have side effects of various levels and intensities. Chemotherapy targets rapidly dividing cancer cells, such as the hair follicles, the mouth, the digestive tract, the nails, and the bone marrow, which can cause multiple side effects. Whether having difficulty with chemo, radiation, or oral medications, reporting and discussing what strategies you can use to be comfortable is vital. Don't wait for your next appointment to make a call!

> If you do nothing else to take care of yourself during treatment, determining the best person to communicate with and how to do so quickly and efficiently will be the most important thing you can do to ensure optimal well-being during your treatment.

I was lucky to find an angel during my treatment at Duke Medical Center. Her name was Felicia, and she managed what they called a triage line for problems or questions that would arise in between treatment. She always called back promptly after my leaving a message and helped me navigate the situation I found myself in. She was proactive in helping me think about managing the days ahead as well. I will always be eternally grateful for her beautiful soul in navigating me through the challenges I faced during chemotherapy. And don't forget that you can have a patient navigator of your own to help you through this process (see Chapter 3: When Someone Is Diagnosed).

#64: Exercise has many therapeutic benefits before, during, and after cancer treatment.

The *American College of Sports Medicine Roundtable on Exercise Guidelines for Cancer Survivors,* published in 2010, reviewed the research around cancer and exercise so that health care teams and survivors could make informed decisions when it came to exercise. Research shows positive benefits for survivors to exercise and stay active before, during, and after treatment, with a few special precautions. New research is continually pointing to significant benefits, so stay tuned to learn more.

Some researchers suggest, for example, that exercise may improve the effects of certain types of therapies while also protecting the cardiovascular system against the harmful effects of these approaches. Answers to these types of questions are currently being investigated.

When exercise is performed that increases heart rate and breathing, such as a brisk walk, we know there are many beneficial, therapeutic effects. Exercise positively impacts almost all of our body's systems at once, much more than any one pill could ever do.

Benefits of Exercise Before and During Treatment

- *Before treatment*: Exercise may reduce stress and anxiety, and strengthen the body to handle what's ahead.
- *During treatment*: Exercise may reduce fatigue, improve quality of life, improve the ability to do daily activities, reduce depression and anxiety, elevate mood, strengthen the immune system, reduce treatment related nausea, improve sleep, may help to minimize the loss of bone and lean body mass and minimize the increase in fat or adipose tissue that often occurs during chemotherapy.

For all people, regardless of cancer status, *avoiding inactivity* is one of the most compelling recommendations ever given by the U.S. Department of Health and Human Services, in my opinion.

Following are the 2008 Physical Activity Guidelines For Americans, included here as a reference. However, it is also important to listen to your body and talk to your doctor before beginning an exercise program. For most people, walking is a safe activity that can be performed throughout treatment, without requiring special supervision. According to the 2008 Physical Activity Guidelines For Americans, adults gain substantial health benefits by doing the following physical activity:

> Cancer survivors should follow the 2008 Physical Activity Guidelines for Americans and avoid inactivity, unless health status, treatment, or disease-related issues call for special modifications.

- Minimum of 150 minutes of *moderate*-intensity aerobic activity spread throughout each week (up to 300 minutes for optimal health benefits)
- *Or:* Minimum of 75 minutes of *vigorous*-intensity aerobic activity spread throughout each week (up to 150 minutes for optimal health benefits)
- *Or:* An equivalent mix of moderate and vigorous intensity aerobic activity
- *And:* Muscle strengthening activities at least two days a week that work all major muscle groups (legs, hips, back, abdomen, chest or shoulders, and arms).

Aerobic activity or cardiovascular activity gets you breathing harder and your heart beating faster. All types of activities count, as long as you're doing them at a *moderate* or *vigorous intensity* for *at least 10 minutes at a time*. You can accumulate them all week long to meet the guidelines.

Definitions

Vigorous-intensity: At this level, you won't be able to say more than a few words without pausing for a breath. Your heart is beating fast. Examples of vigorous effort: Jogging or running, swimming laps, riding a bike fast or on hills, playing singles tennis, playing basketball, heavy gardening (digging, hoeing).

Moderate-intensity: You are working hard enough to raise your heart rate and *break a sweat*. One way to tell is that you'll be able to talk, but not sing the words to your favorite song. Examples of moderate effort: Walking fast, doing water aerobics, riding a bike on level ground, playing doubles tennis, pushing a lawn mower, general gardening (raking), ballroom and line dancing.

Light intensity: Physical activity where your body isn't working hard enough to get your heart rate up or sweat. At this level, you can sing while doing the activity. Examples: Shopping, cooking, doing the laundry, a strolling walk. These activities don't count toward the physical activity guidelines, but are important for overall weight management and daily function.

Muscle strengthening: Activities that work all the different parts of the body—your legs, hips, back, chest, stomach, shoulders, and arms. Work 8 to 10 muscle groups, making sure to do at least 8 to 12 repetitions of each exercise (or 10 to 15 if over 65 or have a chronic condition like arthritis) with a weight or resistance heavy enough to not be able to do another repetition in good form. If you can do more than 12 repetitions, increase the weight. Examples: Lifting weights using machines, dumbbells, resistance bands, or body weight, push-ups on the floor or against the wall, sit-ups, heavy gardening (digging, shoveling).

Special Things to Remember About Your Exercise Program as a Cancer Patient/Survivor

After a Diagnosis/Before Treatment Begins

If you are already an exerciser, keep moving! Doing so may help your body manage stress that comes with a diagnosis *and* may help you handle the treatment better. If new to exercise, start moving as soon as possible. Walking is the easiest activity to do because it involves doing something you already do! Just dedicate five minutes of continual walking and gradually increase a few minutes/day. If unsure, working under the supervision of a trained professional can help you progress safely and confidently.

During Treatment

The old advice used to be to rest and take it easy. Resting is an important part of recovery, but it is important to remain as active *as you are able,* making at least some exercise a priority. Our bodies were designed to move, and when we don't, we experience a lot of negative health conditions, like bone and muscle loss, weight gain, an increase in fatty tissue, and an increase in other health risks. Find the days in your treatment cycle when you feel better. Some survivors report that the day after treatment, when steroids are in their system, can sometimes be a good day for exercise. Find what works for you.

When it comes to strength training, start with low resistance or weights and progress very slowly. Be sure to review the precautions about lymphedema in Chapter 5 and below. Seek assistance in developing a program if you are new to resistance or strength training.

Regular exercisers may need to temporarily take it at a slower pace than normal or break up exercise into smaller increments throughout the day.

Non-exercisers can start with brief slow walks, slowly adding more time.

At the end of the day, don't beat yourself up if you aren't able to be active like you were before treatment. Think about what you *can* do, even if that means light stretching on a given day, or just walking around the house. Focus on the days you will be able to be active.

> Remember that in working toward the physical activity guidelines, it's important to be as active as your condition and physical abilities allow, but some physical activity is better than none at all. Exercise can be accumulated 10 minutes at a time.

Special Precautions

- Always check with your doctor before beginning an exercise program.
- Consider the guidance of a certified exercise professional with special training or certification in cancer and exercise. A physical therapist can also help you regain function, monitor lymphedema, and progress you to further exercise.

- Cancer survivors who have had surgery that involved removing lymph nodes, mastectomy, or radiation may be at risk for developing lymphedema (see Chapter 5: Side Effects You May Not Know About and What You Can Do About Them for detailed prevention measures). Risk may change over time, and occur over a lifetime, due to scarring that develops.
    - ✓ Consult with a lymphedema specialist before beginning an exercise program.
    - ✓ Working too hard or going beyond a typical workout or intensity may trigger or worsen lymphedema.
    - ✓ Exercise should be started gradually, increased cautiously, and stopped for pain or increased swelling or discomfort (and then seek immediate guidance from your specially trained physical therapist/lymphedema specialist or health care provider).
- Conditions that warrant modifications in routine:
    - ✓ Cancer that has spread to the bone: Avoid high-impact exercises.
    - ✓ Low platelets (bleed or bruise easily): Avoid high-impact exercises.
    - ✓ Hemoglobin (red blood count) less than 8.0: Avoid vigorous exercise.
    - ✓ White cell count less than 500: Avoid activities that may increase risk of infections (like swimming or exercising in a gym).
    - ✓ Osteopenia or osteoporosis: Be aware of the risk of fractures and choose activities carefully, possibly limiting or avoiding high risk or high impact exercises/ activities.
- Conditions in which to avoid exercise and seek guidance from a physician:
    - ✓ Fever
    - ✓ Dizziness
    - ✓ Shortness of breath
    - ✓ Chest pain

#65: Nourishing your body with healthy foods will optimize your well-being.

National guidelines for a healthy diet are no different for cancer survivors, but eating a healthy, balanced diet from whole foods (versus supplements) with plenty of fruits and vegetables, whole grains, and lean protein is particularly important to provide energy, help with weight management, and assist in healing from the stresses of treatment. If you need to avoid fresh, raw fruits and vegetables because of neutropenia (low white cell counts), then canned, frozen, and cooked and peeled are good options.

It's not about perfection.

Do not beat yourself up if you are not able to follow through and do all the things you want to do to be healthy during treatment. You will have time for that. I was not "perfect" in my eating or exercise habits during treatment. I could tolerate some things in terms of food, and others I could not. I found myself eating many chicken quesadillas with a lot of cheese. The protein in the chicken, the calcium in the cheese, and the pico de gallo (tomatoes, onions, and cilantro) were all good for me, but the saturated fat and extra calories in the cheese were not the best. However, I found when I ate a meal, I could actually feel energy coming back into my body in a way I had never noticed before. Eating a nourishing meal or snack really served me well and helped with fatigue and overall well-being.

#66: When it comes to eating healthy, start with the basics.

Most people, including survivors, don't eat the *minimum* recommended daily servings of fruits and vegetables, are overweight, and don't exercise. The most basic, first step in staying healthy should be incorporating the minimum guidelines, such as eating fruits and vegetables. In Chapter 7: Optimal Well-Being After Treatment, I've included those guidelines.

Within that healthy diet, you can make optimal choices to support your body's immune system and healing ability. In *Anticancer, A New Way of Life* by David Servan-Schreiber, he talks about his own cancer and how he learned about the body's natural cancer fighting abilities, what makes cancer cells in our bodies thrive, and what inhibits them. After reading this book, you'll most likely never look at what you put into your body as inconsequential. Always remember: every meal or snack is an opportunity to improve your health and build your immune system or take away from it.

When looking for a registered dietitian (RD) in private practice, or within an organization, there is a new certification for dietitians working in the field of oncology, called a certified specialist in oncology nutrition (CSO). The Oncology Nutrition Dietetic Practice Group is a group within the American Dietetic Association, and the group has worked with the Commission on Dietetic Registration to create a board certification credential for registered dietitians in oncology nutrition. Even if a CSO dietitian is not near you, finding an RD who has some experience with cancer survivors will be a benefit to you.

#67: Supplements, antioxidants, herbs, and unproven diets may cause harm.

When it comes to nutrition and cancer, no subject garners more interest, yet it's an area where great misinformation abounds. A diagnosis can become a catalyst for making positive lifestyle changes, including better nutrition and eating habits. Yet, it is also a time when many question the foods they've eaten in the past that might have been a cause for their disease. That search for answers can sometimes lead people to unproven diets or supplements with claims of a cure that might actually cause more harm.

For example, taking antioxidant or herbal supplements during treatment may make treatments less effective and reduce survival, as they may protect tumor cells (while also protecting healthy cells), according to published, randomized research. Always talk to your oncologist about any supplements you may be taking that could impact your treatment outcomes. *Remember: no known dietary supplements have been proven to treat or cure cancer.*

I know during my treatment, I had people from all walks of life (even strangers) tell me what I needed to do. There are many myths, misconceptions, and even lies about what will help you. While some of the advice may be spot on and accurate, it's important to know where the information came from. Is someone selling a product that "mainstream medicine" doesn't accept? Be wary. It doesn't mean that there may not be some truth, but what it does mean is that there may not be solid, peer reviewed, published research on the subject. If there is not, why risk it? Everything we put in our mouths can have a medicinal effect, acting like medicines (prescription or over the counter). *Natural* doesn't necessarily mean safe. Most drugs are made from something in nature.

Question the "science" or "research" behind a product or recommendation that sounds too good to be true:
- Has it been published and peer reviewed (others in same field) in a reputable journal?
- Has research been done on human beings other than in a Petri dish?
- Was the research done around the specific claim they are making?
- Can you get a copy of it?
- When a doctor is associated with the product, are the person's background and credentials relevant to the type of research or product?
- What does your oncologist think about it?

Your life is too important to risk natural methods that have not been proven, so be wary!

#68: Many things can be done to help you cope with and minimize nausea.

Sometimes nausea and appetite for certain foods can get in the way of eating healthy and getting essential nutrients. Rather than throw in the towel when not quite meeting healthy guidelines, give yourself a break, eat as healthily as you are able, and seek help. Most cancer centers have printed materials with information and tips for good nutrition during cancer treatment as well as a registered dietitian on staff who can provide special assistance or answer questions. They can make suggestions to help you find alternatives if a certain group of foods are not palatable. For example, instead of red meat, fish, or poultry for protein, you could substitute legumes (beans), peanut butter, eggs, yogurt, milk, or cheese. Online sources are also plentiful, and survivors can also go to reputable sites that are referenced at the end of the book.

With the right medication, nausea and vomiting can be minimized, if not eliminated in most patients. In addition, other tools can help. One study at the University of California at San Francisco showed that 20 minutes of moderate exercise, three times per week, significantly reduced nausea intensity.

Be proactive in working with your team to get the most aggressive medication protocol from the very beginning. It is easier to keep nausea away than to make it go away once you have it. Don't wait until you are nauseated to take the medicine.

Ginger has been used for centuries to minimize nausea associated with other conditions. An NCI funded trial showed that ginger helped prevent or reduce nausea during chemotherapy when it was taken with anti-nausea drugs. The most effective doses were either 500 mg or 1000 mg taken during the first day of chemotherapy. Using a quarter or half teaspoon twice a day of grated ginger is easy to use and has not shown harm and may actually help. Before taking any supplement, be sure to talk to your doctor.

Other Tips

- Eat dry food like crackers, toast, or dry cereal.
- Eat small amounts of food throughout the day (every two to three hours).
- Stay upright after meals to keep acid reflux from aggravating nausea.
- Avoid strong smells when possible.
- Switch to cold entrées when needed (warm food tends to have stronger smells, causing more aversion to the food)

Distraction is another great tool for taking your mind off how you are feeling. Whether it's work, a walk outside, a funny video, a phone conversation with a friend, or a puzzle, staying busy can help to distract you from thinking about how you feel.

#69: Staying hydrated with plenty of water allows your body to do the work it needs to do.

Some medications can be dehydrating and will contribute to constipation. If water tastes bad, find low-calorie options, like tea, coffee (decaf preferred), or other ways of flavoring water (lemons, limes, etc.). I've coached a lot of people who hated water to just keep it around and take little sips throughout the day. They not only consumed eight glasses in a day, but started losing weight because they substituted water for sugary drinks/juice. Liquid calories add up, so limit sugar-filled drinks that may contribute to growing your waistline.

#70: Balancing the expected roller coaster of emotions and stress with strategies and support will help to minimize the downsides of cancer.

According to Joel Siegel, the movie critic, his friend Gilda Radner, an original cast member of *Saturday Night Live* who died of ovarian cancer, used to say, "If it wasn't for the downside, having cancer would be the best thing and everyone would want it." The gift of the kindness of humanity and the realization of what really matters in life are some of the most special gifts to receive from cancer. However, cancer and its treatment is not always a road paved with pretty flowers and sunshine.

It is normal for emotions to run the gamut after a life-threatening diagnosis. Everyone's response will vary, depending on a person's particular diagnosis and the treatment plan that will follow. The more aggressive the treatment, the more life-altering a diagnosis will be, and thus the emotions to follow because of that impact. It is always a "Whoa, wow, I can't believe this is happening" moment, but many factors will impact a person's level of response.

So often, everyone is bent on keeping us positive, when the reality often feels much different. A positive mindset is also important, but feeling the sadness and loss helps us process what is happening instead of ignoring or denying it. As human beings, we were born with the ability to have emotions, to feel and react to life as it happens. It's important to allow whatever feelings you have to be felt. Expressing them in a safe setting, whether it's to a family member, friend, or support professional, is crucial to our mental health. Stress, anxiety, grief, and feelings of depression are normal responses. However, if the feelings of sadness become persistent and not balanced with positive emotion, it's time to talk to your doctor and seek support.

Balancing the downside with positive emotions in a deliberate, planned manner can help mediate, brighten the journey, and cultivate a greater sense of well-being. Finding emotional balance within the storm of treatment may take a little forethought and planning. Some of the many strategies include: meditation, yoga, tai chi, support groups, talking to a social worker, prayer, regular visits with friends on the phone or in person, staying involved in activities that keep you connected or feeling purposeful, regular physical activity or exercise, taking care of yourself and setting boundaries, keeping a gratitude journal, and many more.

I recommend building a portfolio of some of these positive ideas, activities, or experiences that make you smile, laugh, bring peace, or have gratitude. Whether it is a physical file folder or a folder on your computer, having a place to go with pictures, ideas, reminders, or other items is extremely helpful to remind us when we have forgotten. It could be pictures of loved ones, a funny comic strip, a link to a YouTube video, a card someone has written, an email, a list of funny movies or TV shows to watch, or a life-giving inspirational event, poem, or saying. It could also be a list of the things that bring you energy so you will remember to include them in your day. It's like creating a treasure chest and arsenal for all the things in life that make you feel joy, satisfaction, or gratitude, when the not-so-great days come. It's the days when the sun isn't shining that having prompts to remind us of what is right in our world that is invaluable. I have a friend who actually took a folder like this to chemotherapy to keep her spirits high.

Positive psychologist Barbara Fredrickson talks about the ideal balance of positive to negative emotions for all people (not just cancer), as a 3:1 ratio of positive to negative emotions. Her research found that for every negative thought, we should try to balance with three positive emotions, to thrive as human beings.

I found gratitude to be one of the easiest and most helpful positive emotions to use to shift my mood during my treatment, because I could do it no matter where I was or what I was doing. I didn't need to be "doing" anything. Being alive, waking up to a new day, and appreciating the kindness shown by strangers always lifted my spirits and even gratitude for the ability to walk. I will never again take for granted the ability and energy to go to a grocery store and shop for my groceries, which was very difficult at times during my treatment.

I remember one day, lying in bed and writhing in pain. As it came in waves, I would have moments of respite. In those moments, I was so grateful for it to stop that I would literally say "Thank you" out loud. Many times, I would feel down and impatient, thinking about how life was passing me by. In letting my mind go to thoughts of gratitude and being present at that moment, I could calm my mind.

When we are feeling good, it's easy to be grateful and happy. It's harder when life isn't so great that challenge appears. Having a plan in place for self-care with ideas for feeling better is enormously helpful—cancer or no cancer.

#71: Setting boundaries to support your health and well-being will minimize stress.

As a wellness coach, I've found that many women seek to please and take care of others, often to the detriment of their own health and well-being. While one of the most beautiful attributes of a woman is her ability to nurture and care for others, when it comes at the cost of her own health, it's not so beautiful. Self-care requires setting boundaries—boundaries that allow for taking care of our spirits, minds, and bodies. When we do that, we will be able be our best for those we care about.

Stress is abundant when we are burning the candles at both ends. Treatment is a perfect time to begin thinking about what you need to be your best and then following through with it. People will respect and honor what you say you need, because they want to be helpful. Putting your health first during this time has the potential to last a lifetime.

Setting boundaries will look different for everyone. It may mean saying no to obligations or requests such as babysitting grandchildren, making dinner each night, volunteering, cleaning the house, taking phone calls around the clock, or other activities that fill our lives.

It becomes profoundly important to ask, where is my limited energy best spent right now? How can I support my body to get through treatment and thrive? What do I need to let go of, and/or what is not serving me well right now?

One of my clients was overwhelmed with friends calling her. She wanted to talk to friends, but she valued the time with her young child and was very stressed about time away from her. Her solution was to set specific hours when she would visit with friends on the phone. She sent out an email to everyone announcing what she was doing. Friends respected her time and understood, even though she was a little worried they might not.

I found I was especially sensitive to negative energy around me during treatment. Arguing, complaining loudly, or other negative behavior felt damaging. I think at such a vulnerable and weakened state, I actually felt it much more strongly than I would have otherwise. I asked for what I needed or set boundaries so I was not around it. It is amazing what happens when you ask for what you need.

Contrary to popular myths, no evidence is available to support the claim that stress can cause a recurrence, but our reaction to stress can certainly impact the healthy behaviors we choose to engage in, which *will* impact our longevity.

#72: Taking time to look good will make you feel better.

The American Cancer Society has a program called Look Good…Feel Better®, which holds classes to show women some of the things they can do to look their best during treatment. The program exists because looking our best makes us feel better and impacts our outlook and well-being. When we look better, we *do* feel better. Let's face it; chemotherapy is not a prescribed beauty regimen. However, we can do certain things to optimize our beauty during chemotherapy.

First, we all know that beauty comes from the inside and shines outward. It is what matters most. One woman told me during my treatment that there was something about a woman undergoing treatment that made them beautiful and shine. She couldn't put her finger on it, but she believed it with her heart and soul. Was it their vulnerability? Renewed appreciate for life? Who knows? I know I didn't feel pretty, but I appreciate her saying so. But, we can do many things to feel beautiful both inside and out during treatment, aside from all we've already talked about.

Hair and Eyebrows

A woman's hair is highly valued in our society, and losing it—even if temporarily—can be devastating to many. Finding a style that suits you is important, whether finding wigs, special scarves, or fun hats that make you feel pretty. If you are one of the lucky ones who can sport a bald head with confidence, go for it! I wore long scarves tied in a bow to the side with a hat on top. I did get a wig or two, but I did not like them enough to wear them often. Many cancer centers and non-profits have access to low- or no-cost services for a wig or head covering.

One day, this side effect could be a thing of the past. A promising new therapy is being studied that has worked for some people called "cold cap" therapy, in which ice packs are placed on the head during chemotherapy. It's an intense process that would require support from the health care team. However, because no longitudinal studies are available at this time, most physicians are not quite ready to support it for fear that cancer cells might not be killed that are present in the scalp, but stay tuned!

When hair grows back in, it will probably be a bit different than it was before. During radiation, my hair grew back in a grayish hue, kinky and curly—something I had was not fond of. If you find the same happening to you, hair stylists can offer tips to optimize your beauty and style it in a way that works for you. I went through many hair products, working to find the best solution as my hair grew back. The good news is that eventually, for most, it goes back to its original state.

Makeup

Makeup is an essential part of pulling together new looks, from no hair to new short hair, that will work for you. Learning to use makeup to optimize my appearance was helpful, even though I had always worn makeup. Even if you are not one who wears it, a few little items can give you a lift. I found a makeup counter that helped me with drawing natural looking eyebrows. I had a few scattered hairs that helped guide me, using a special eyebrow brush and light powder. Eyebrows frame the face, and when they aren't there, we don't look like ourselves. Makeup counters have all kinds of experiences with people who have permanent alopecia (hair loss) or other conditions and can help you with tips to get through. Even if you don't buy any makeup there, you can use their advice when you get home.

Clothes

I'm a big believer in dressing for the day, no matter what. Even if you don't see anyone, it starts the day with purpose. Dressing in clothes that make you feel good or pretty is an added boost that might feel like pampering, but why not? You deserve it! I've never seen anyone who dressed in their best and favorite clothes slump their shoulders and frown. Why put something on that you don't like? If money is an issue, go to thrift stores and find some clothes that make you smile. Believe me, I've done that on more than one occasion. I did gain some weight during this time and bought a few pieces of clothing that I used during treatment. They felt good at the time, and later I was happy to get rid of them, as they reminded me of some not-so-great moments. But when possible, dress for feeling your best, even if it's a silky nightgown and robe!

#73: You can optimize energy by understanding the specific challenges of cancer-related fatigue and sleep disruption and having a plan to address them.

Managing fatigue and sleep disruption are two of the most common concerns of survivors, according to the Breast Cancer Registry. Quality of life during, and even years after, treatment can be impacted by the side effects of fatigue and problems with sleep.

Fatigue and sleep habits may seem related, but are separate. I've put them together because disrupted sleep can compound problems with cancer-related fatigue (CRF). The type of cancer-related fatigue experienced with chemotherapy and radiation is much different than being tired, where sleep or rest delivers relief. The exact reason for cancer-related fatigue is being investigated, but multiple factors could contribute, including the cancer itself, pain, medications, stress, depression, anemia, decreased nutrition, and many others.

A finite amount of energy is available with CRF. I describe it like being a battery-operated Energizer® bunny. For me, when the energy was used up on a given day, it was over, and was not replenished with a rest or nap.

It is important to try to assess with your health care team what the cause(s) may be in your situation, because another underlying cause could be treated. Keeping a log for a week of sleep patterns and energy levels throughout the day may be helpful for your team to assist in identifying other possible causes.

SUGGESTIONS FOR MANAGING CANCER-RELATED FATIGUE

- Prioritize and simplify what matters most to accomplish in a given day and what could be delegated. Some days it might mean just getting dressed and getting to a doctor's appointment. I was always surprised at what energy it took to get myself showered and ready. Many days, it was a major accomplishment.
- Conserve energy and pace yourself throughout the day, understanding that your energy stores are limited.
- Learn to let go of things you think *have* to be done, and allow others to help with routine chores (things like grocery shopping, cooking, or cleaning).
- Keep a list of things that will give you energy, and make sure to include them in your day to balance energy-draining tasks you might have to do. Some ideas of energy-giving activities: talking to a close friend; watching a favorite movie/TV show; arts and crafts; listening to music, singing, or playing an instrument; an outdoor walk in the woods or park; exercise; reading a good book or magazine.
- Though it seems counterintuitive, exercising regularly with the kind of exercise that gets the heart rate up, even for a short period of time, can minimize CRF. Being

careful to gradually progress the amount of time and intensity is important (but without overdoing it), as noted previously. It can also help with anxiety, depression, stiffness, minor aches and pain, and improve many other health conditions.

- Drink plenty of water or other fluids. Lack of hydration will contribute to fatigue in anyone.
- Eat foods that contribute to positive energy and health, such as fruits, vegetables, whole grains, and lean protein.

DIFFICULTY WITH FALLING AND STAYING ASLEEP

Difficulty with falling and staying asleep is one of the most frustrating side effects survivors experience because of its impact across all areas of one's life. Sleep plays a major role in healing our bodies.

Before cancer, I never had trouble getting a good night's sleep. Going through immediate menopause and experiencing chemotherapy (and related drugs) impacted my sleep during treatment and years after. During treatment, I was given a low-dose anti-anxiety drug (Ativan®) to go to sleep, which I became reliant on. I have to say that I was upset when they wouldn't refill the prescription, but I understood why. Staying on that particular drug for any length of time would cause another host of problems. Staying asleep was difficult for years, but I wish I had known all the tricks of getting a good night's sleep in order to stack the odds in my favor.

A good night's sleep is critical to your health. Learning to optimize the energy you have to start the day, even when that energy may be limited, is vital. According to the Harvard Women's Health Watch, there are six reasons to make sure we get enough sleep (regardless of cancer status):

- *Learning and memory:* Sleeping helps the brain process new information to memory. With cognitive impact from treatment being a concern, survivors need all the help we can get.
- *Metabolism and weight:* Our appetite is impacted when we don't get enough sleep, altering levels of hormones that affect our appetites.
- *Safety:* We are more likely to make mistakes or errors in judgment when we don't get enough sleep.
- *Mood:* Who isn't a bit cranky with too little sleep?
- *Cardiovascular health:* Sleep disorders have been linked to high blood pressure, increased stress hormone levels, and irregular heartbeat.
- *Disease:* Immune function is improved with a good night's sleep, and cancer may be linked to not enough sleep.

Following good sleep hygiene and sleep habits as perfectly as possible will optimize a chance at quality sleep. Following them may not make for a perfect night's sleep, but will at least give you the best baseline to start from and minimize problems. I think of looking at them in the same way as other health habits that are important as we get older. What we could get away with when we were young doesn't work anymore.

Remember, even when doing everything "perfectly," a good night's sleep may still be challenging. A physician may prescribe medications for sleeping in the short term, but they can't be relied on indefinitely. Developing healthy sleep routines and habits can help minimize the disruption that is inevitable.

Overall, most research shows the need for adults to get at least seven to eight hours of sleep each night to maximize the benefits that occur when we sleep. Building the intention to get a good night's sleep starts with setting the time aside and making it a priority. If six hours has been the norm, gradually increase the time you intend to sleep by 15-minute increments. It is amazing what our bodies will do when we make the intention a part of our health routine.

Habits That Support a Good Night's Sleep

During the Day

- First thing in the morning, open the curtains to expose natural light to reinforce the body's sleep-wake cycle.
- Avoid naps during the day whenever possible because they will impact evening sleep. Resting is different than napping and is fine. If a nap is unavoidable, a "catnap" of no more than 10 to 15 minutes mid-afternoon can give needed relief.
- Avoid anything with caffeine (coffee, chocolate, tea, etc) after 3:00 (or an earlier time if that is your body's response). Though chocolate may not have a lot of caffeine, if you are sensitive to caffeine, it can make a difference.

In the Evening

- Avoid exercise within three hours before bedtime, but if unavoidable (because exercise is so important to health and well-being), do it as early in the evening as possible. Exercise speeds up the body's metabolism and raises the body's temperature, working against the gradual slowdown that naturally occurs in the evening toward bedtime. That being said, some research shows that exercising five to six hours before bedtime will raise the body's temperature, but then after four or five hours take it lower than it would have been if you had not exercised. This decrease in body temperature would maximize exercise's beneficial effects on sleep. So walking at 5 p.m. might work if going to bed between 10 and 11 p.m. Timing is everything!
- Avoid heavy, high-fat evening meals, but include ones high in carbohydrates with a medium amount of protein to help you relax (serotonin from the carbs). High-protein meals are better earlier in the day with evening meals containing more complex carbohydrates such as fruits, vegetables, and whole grains or pasta.

- Avoid eating at least two to three hours before bedtime because eating food speeds up the body's metabolism.
- If evening snacks are inevitable, take advantage of foods that will help you sleep. The best foods will have a nice balance of complex carbohydrates, calcium, and a small amount of protein. Foods that have tryptophan (a sleep-inducing amino acid) as well as calcium (helps the brain use tryptophan to manufacture melatonin) will give the body that extra boost to induce sleep, if eaten one hour before bedtime (it takes about that long for the foods to reach the brain).
  - ✓ Examples: Whole-grain cereal with milk, peanut butter sandwich and milk, fruit and cheese
  - ✓ Tryptophan-containing foods: All dairy, soy, seafood, meat, poultry, whole grains, beans, rice, hummus, lentils, eggs, sesame and sunflower seeds

Routines and Environment

- An hour or two before bedtime, start dimming the lights and winding down, doing activities that are not extremely stimulating.
- Develop a routine in the last hour before bedtime that will support your body recognizing it is winding down for sleep. Sample routines might be getting into pajamas, brushing teeth, a warm bath, stretching, reading a book/magazine (easy read, not stimulating), or writing in a journal. Meditation, prayer, gratitude exercises, or listening to calm, soothing music just before bed will calm the body and soul for sleep.
- Keep the bedroom dark with blackout shades, if possible, covering any LED lights in the room. A dark room not only supports a good night's sleep, but helps the body produce melatonin (only produced by the body in darkness) which *may* help reduce risk for cancers, impact weight management, and other disease. It is produced by the pineal gland, deep in the brain. Recent research has shown that blindness is a protective factor for breast cancer. Countries that generate the most light at night have the highest incidence of breast cancer. Shift work has been associated with higher cancer incidence as well.
- Get to bed by 10 p.m., when the body's natural rhythms make it easiest to fall asleep.
- Keep regular bedtime and wake-up hours to support the sleep-wake cycle. It is not possible to "catch up" on sleep on the weekends.
- When possible, sleep on a comfortable, supportive mattress with a good pillow.
- Adjust the thermostat at night to be cooler while sleeping.
- Wear an eye pillow if you are sensitive to light that might wake you up.
- Minimize or avoid activities in the bedroom other than sleep and sex (like television) so the room and the bed equate to sleep.

Waking During the Night and Getting Back to Sleep

During periods of physical and emotional stress, it is not uncommon for sleep to be interrupted. In addition, hot flashes can interfere with sleep by causing night sweats that are disruptive. Pre-menopausal women who go through sudden and severe menopause with treatment (as well as menopausal women who are already experiencing this) are particularly impacted.

- Wear breathable fabrics.
- Keep a fan beside the bed to turn toward you when waking with a flash. The white noise can be an added benefit to help you get back to sleep. This is the most important part of my coping, as quick cooling allowed me to go back into my slumber.
- Keep the room temperature cooler at night when possible.

Falling Back to Sleep After Being Awakened

- Use breathing techniques to relax your body. Instead of thinking "I've got to get back to sleep," think "I'm just going to breathe, rest, and relax my body."
- Keep a relaxation tape, mp3, or other recording near your bedside that will help you get back to sleep. Many are available on the market (and even free versions online) that can help you through a progressive relaxation process.
- Use visualization that creates a focus on something like counting sheep, praying for others, remembering a dream, or other focus that won't engage you in thinking about details of your life.
- Get up if 20 to 30 minutes has passed and go to another room in the dimmest light possible and do a boring task or read something that isn't interesting to you.
- Avoid looking at the clock, and hide it if you can.
- If you know you are only sleeping six hours at a time, go to bed later. Yes, it's better to sleep longer, but if your body is not cooperating, it may add to your frustration to wake up too early and not be able to go back to sleep.

Lifestyle Habits

- Studies have shown that people who exercise sleep better. Exercise on most days, developing the highest level of fitness possible. Regular exercise helps the body's systems do what they are supposed to do. Our bodies were designed to move, and when they do not, none of the systems work optimally.
- Eat a balanced diet, including healthy carbohydrates, like a variety of fruits, vegetables, and whole grains during the day.

#74: Building a team of support professionals will enhance optimal well-being during and after treatment.

In Chapter 8: Giving, Receiving, and Seeking Support, I address the important role of friends and family in supporting optimal well-being. In addition, building a team of support professionals can help enormously. Most of the professionals can also be helpful for the time after treatment.

The following services can sometimes be covered by insurance, offered free by an organization, be a fee-for-service, or included as a benefit under health savings accounts. If there is a fee and it is not reimbursed by insurance, gifts from friends and family can sometimes be an option if resources are limited. I know I've had people come to me wanting to pay for a friend or loved one wanting to be coached.

Patient navigator: Mentioned in Chapter 3: When Someone Is Diagnosed a professional who can help you navigate treatment and beyond is a must-have. I highly recommend www.NavigateCancerFoundation.org for an oncology nurse navigator who is independent of a cancer center or institution. Because the definitions of navigators vary, it doesn't hurt to have more than one. For example, some may be based on helping you navigate your health care system in particular, while another might be a peer navigator (another survivor trained to support you).

Social worker/counselor/psychologist: Many centers and non-profit cancer organizations have social workers who have specific experience and training in counseling cancer patients and survivors. Sometimes, talking to a professional who understands the challenges you are facing can alleviate stress by helping you manage and sort through the variety of emotions you might be experiencing. Even one or two visits can make a huge difference. CancerCare (www.cancercare.org) has oncology social workers available via phone at no charge.

Support groups can also be helpful in navigating the experience of cancer. They can be online, by phone, or in person. They connect people experiencing similar challenges, offering a chance to share advice and tips, talk openly about concerns in a safe place, and help you feel less isolated.

Registered dietitian: A dietitian can help in determining a strategy to manage nutrition-related side effects, or determining your survivorship eating plan. Find a dietitian with oncology experience by searching the American Dietetic Association website (www.eatright.org) or calling their 800 number. The American Cancer Society also has a "dietitian on-call" program.

Physical therapist: A therapist trained in working with breast cancer survivors can help you rehabilitate from surgery, manage side effects from treatment that impact function, and help you monitor any risk of lymphedema.

Cancer exercise trainer: Cancer exercise trainers can help you develop an exercise routine to safely maintain or progress your fitness level. They can help you develop one at home or work with you individually. Though a certified personal trainer can be found through an online search, some cancer centers have cancer rehab programs. Medically based fitness or wellness centers (affiliated with a hospital) are also great places to find qualified professionals, as are integrative medicine centers.

The American College of Sports Medicine and the American Cancer Society have a fitness certification for professionals working with cancer patients and survivors called ACSM Cancer Exercise Trainer or CET. Go to www.ACSM.org/certification to find a certified professional near you. Some YMCAs, community non-profits, or universities have special exercise programs for cancer survivors that can be beneficial as well.

Integrative medicine programs: Sometimes cancer centers have a connection with a center for integrative medicine. Those centers house many of these professionals, but also have other complementary (working alongside and with traditional treatment) interventions such as yoga, stress-reduction classes, acupuncture, massage, and other mind-body healing techniques that can be tremendously beneficial.

Wellness coach: A certified wellness coach with a professional background in health and fitness can help you think through what will optimize your well-being and develop a plan that will work for you, incorporating all the things that have been discussed in this and other chapters. They can help you learn what you need to know about healthy eating and exercise as well as partner with you to develop sustainable lifestyle habits.

I was a co-investigator and coach looking at the longitudinal (long-term) impact and benefits of wellness coaching for cancer survivors after treatment. In the first published study around wellness coaching as a single intervention (as well as for cancer survivors), we found statistically significant results showing that wellness coaching reduced anxiety, depression, improved quality of life, and supported sustainable lifestyle changes, one year after the intervention ended. Though it was a small study and further research needs to be done, wellness coaching with the right coach may be exactly what survivors need to build and sustain healthier, happier lives after a diagnosis of cancer.

When looking for a health, fitness, or wellness coach, the American College of Sports Medicine endorses those certified by Wellcoaches Corporation. Coaches must have credentials and a background in one area of health care in order to be certified. I have a personal bias that coaches who are also certified by ACSM or other nationally recognized fitness certifications are the most qualified to help people with exercise, weight loss, and lifestyle changes. Having a cancer and exercise certification and/or other experience in the field of oncology is important. However, an oncology nurse or dietitian trained as a wellness coach might also be an added bonus during treatment, transitioning to a health and fitness professional trained as a wellness coach after treatment ends.

The research above was based on my program for coaching cancer survivors. For more information go to: www.HealthyandFitAfterCancer.com. Coaching is primarily done by phone, so there are no geographical boundaries.

Chapter References

The Cancer Support Community
www.csc.BreastCancerRegistry.org.

D'Andrea, G. (2005). Use of antioxidants during chemotherapy and radiotherapy should be avoided. *CA Cancer J Clin*. 55: 319–321.

Doyle, C., Kushi, L.H., Byers, T., Courneya, K.S., Demark-Wahnefried, W., Grant, B., McTiernan, A., Rock, C.L., Thompson, C., Gansler, T., & Andrews, K.S. (2006). Nutrition and physical activity during and after cancer treatment: an American cancer society guide for informed choices. *CA: A Cancer Journal for Clinicians*. 56: 323–353.

Demark-Wahnefried, W., Peterson, B.L., Winer, E.P., Marks, L., Aziz, N., Marcom, P.K., Blackwell, K., & Rimer, B.K. (2001). Changes in weight, body composition and factors influencing energy balance among premenopausal breast cancer patients receiving adjuvant chemotherapy. *Journal of Clinical Oncology*. 19: 2381–2389.

Demark-Wahnefried, W., Winer, E.P., & Rimer, B.K. (1993). Why women gain weight with adjuvant chemotherapy for breast cancer. *Journal of Clinical Oncology*. 11: 1418–1429.

Demark-Wahnefried, W., Hars, V., Conaway, M., Havlin, K., Rimer, B., McElveen, G., & Winer, E. (1997). Reduced rates of metabolism and decreased physical activity in breast cancer patients receiving adjuvant chemotherapy. *American Journal of Clinical Nutrition*. 65: 1495–1501.

Doyle, C., Kushi, L.H., Byers, T., et al (2006). Nutrition and physical activity during and after cancer treatment: An American Cancer Society guide for informed choices. *CA Cancer J Clin*. 56(6): 323–353.

Exercise Is Medicine
www.ExerciseIsMedicine.org.

Flynn-Evans, E.E., Stevens, R.G., Tabandeh, H., Schernhammer, E.S., & Lockley, S.W. (2009). Total visual blindness is protective against breast cancer. *Cancer Causes Control*. 20(9): 1753–1756.

Lawenda, B.D., et al (2008). Should supplemental antioxidant administration be avoided during chemotherapy and radiation therapy? *J Natl Cancer Inst*. Jun 4, 100(11): 773–783.

Lee, J., Dodd, M.J., Dibble, S.L. & Abrams, D.I. (2008). Nausea at the end of adjuvant cancer treatment in relation to exercise during treatment in patients with breast cancer. *Oncol Nurs Forum*. Sept., 35(5): 830–835.

Morey, M.C., Snyder, D.C., Sloane, R., Cohen, H.J., Peterson, B., Hartman, T., Miller, P.E., Mitchell, D., & Demark-Wahnefried, W. (2009). Effects of home-based diet and exercise on functional outcomes among older, overweight long-term cancer survivors. RENEW: A randomized controlled trial. *JAMA*. 301: 1883–1891.

Rock, C.L. & Demark-Wahnefried W. (2002). Nutrition and survival after the diagnosis of breast cancer: a review of the evidence. *Journal of Clinical Oncology*. 20: 3302–3316.

Schmitz, K., Ahmed, R.L., Troxel, A., et al. (2009). Weight lifting in women with breast cancer-related lymphedema. *N Engl J Med*. 361: 664–673.

Schmitz, K.H. (2010). American College of Sports Medicine Roundtable on Exercise Guidelines for Cancer Survivors. *Medicine & Science in Sports & Exercise*. July, 42(7): 1409–1426.

7

Optimal Well-Being
After Treatment

In writing this book, I passed my seventh anniversary (or "cancer-versary") of my diagnosis. I never gave the day much notice in the past, but it was always in the back of my mind. This year, it fell at a time when I was writing and thinking deeply about my experiences. April 12 is the day that I got the infamous call, and is a date that falls in the middle of spring, a time of hope and renewal. That was a year where my hopes and dreams took a backseat for a moment.

Spring was also the time when treatment ended, but this time I was filled with feelings of hope and optimism. Here in North Carolina, it is one of the most beautiful times of year with azaleas and dogwood trees in bloom. The weather is warm, and all living things come out from under their winter blanket, with birds singing and soft green leaves pushing out from their buds.

The Duke Cancer Patient Support Program gave me a picture of a yellow jonquil pushing through the snow with a quote beneath it that read: "In the midst of winter, I finally learned that there was in me an invincible summer. —Albert Camus." It signified the inner strength one finds in the winters of life and that after that darkness, we emerge with great hope for living, and living fully.

What I didn't know was that this spring would carry a mixed bag of emotions and experiences. In spite of the excitement of treatment being over, recovery was not an overnight process. I was tired and weak. I had new feelings I was unaccustomed to. I was not the strong person people kept telling me I was. My confidence in myself had been eroded somehow, and I experienced anxiety in a form that was entirely new to me. What was this feeling in the pit of my stomach? Who was I? What was this about?

What I've learned is that I was in "survival mode" during treatment. I had been surviving and holding it together for myself as well as everyone around me. I wasn't consciously aware of the feelings that my body had betrayed me, but now I was. I had invested so much into prevention that it felt as if the rug and all I knew to be true was literally pulled out from under me.

I was discovering what this new place was: my new reality. I would have to learn to live with uncertainty that cancer could return. They could not say I was "cured" as in some types of cancers. I would have to learn that taking care of myself didn't necessarily mean disease would never come, but I could reduce its chances. I would learn that recovery would take a lot of time. I was reassessing my priorities and what really mattered to me. One minute I was excited and hopeful, and the next I was filled with anxiety.

All of this uncertainty and questioning, combined with a weakened body and foggy brain, made some situations and circumstances more difficult than they might have been. I was asked to be a keynote speaker at an annual event for the Duke Cancer Patient Support Program. They were also giving me the Jonquil Award. Past speakers had been famous and beloved. No one knew me, and worse yet, who was I to receive this or speak to this huge audience? Anxiety filled every part of my being for the months leading up to it. I was honored, yet not the same confident woman I once was. About the same time, a highly respected colleague delivered information they felt would help me since I was reassessing my life and priorities. The information was insulting, impacted my reputation in my field, was based on lies, and I was told I couldn't defend, address, or confront the untruths. Further, it was delivered with no empathy or understanding. I was devastated and confused. I felt kicked when I was down. In their defense, they had no way of knowing how vulnerable and weak I truly was. I was excited about my new life, but I was not invincible.

Women going back to work and the fullness of what their lives entail may be subject to similar expectations. "Okay, you've been out for awhile, it's over … let's get her going again!" Survivors may jump back in trying to do it all and work hard to catch up for time lost. Because I have coached many women after treatment, I know that what I experienced was not unique. It looks different on everyone, but there is no doubt it is a time of vulnerability, reassessment, and recovery.

I lead with this story, because it's important to know that this time of transition is normal. You will not suddenly feel back to normal after one week. What does it take to recover from cancer treatment and be stronger than ever? A realization and understanding that we have the ability to impact our recovery, that we can take charge of our health and well-being. What else? Patience. Focus. Time. A plan. Determination. Support. Rest. Exercise. Sleep. Good nutrition. Healthy weight. Healthy lifestyle. And stronger than ever doesn't necessarily mean back to the same person you once were, because that is unlikely, but it can mean better and stronger in different ways. How long will it take? It depends. It was years before I felt back to normal, whatever that is, but I didn't have the support I'm offering here. I had no one to tell me what I needed to do to recover!

And though survivors are most concerned about reducing their risk for recurrence, we need to be concerned about our risk for other diseases. The number-one killer of cancer survivors is still heart disease, as it is for most women! Developing healthy habits helps us all the way around.

We can do much to control our health and well-being in spite of bumps that will inevitably come our way. And yes, there will be bumps. Side effects from treatment impacted my recovery many, many times. Sometimes, I felt like I could never catch a break.

Experiencing adversity in any form can break us or make us stronger. While you might feel broken at times, resiliency comes from life's storms. We develop a new appreciation for the simple, good things in life that make us able to focus on what matters most. We learn skills that will see us through future storms, because life is certain to be filled with highs and lows. We grow as human beings and have a renewed empathy for others, especially those living with illness, pain, or chronic diseases. In fact, we can learn to flourish in a way we never have before, bringing renewed purpose, meaning, and appreciation for all things good and right in the world. Science calls it post-traumatic growth!

While it may be one step forward and two steps back at times, what matters is that you are moving forward, one little step at a time. It may also be that your recovery is smooth and steady with few bumps. That is my greatest wish for you!

#75: It will take time to recover, so be patient.

When treatment ended, I assumed that I would quickly regain my prior health and well-being. In fact, about a month or so after radiation ended, I remember talking to a nurse, concerned that I was not regaining my energy and that it had been a month. Her tone of voice let me know I was being a little unrealistic as she told me it would take time. How much time? It depended and was individual. In hindsight, it was silly to think that after the year of aggressive treatment, my body would suddenly be back to normal. After having the flu for a week or two, it takes time to regain strength. Why would I think that after such trauma, it would only take a month?

As you can probably guess, my biggest challenge was patience. I wanted my health back right away. Most of the survivors I coach after treatment ends share that impatience, and are often reluctant to let those around them know that they are still recovering. We want to believe we will be back to normal as soon as treatment is over.

#76: Communicating with others about recovery may ease your transition after treatment.

When treatment ends, there is an opportunity to focus on regaining strength and vitality. When those who are around understand that it is a process and will take time, the more likely support will continue to be there for you. Be as open and honest as possible, asking for support when you need it, and set boundaries that will allow you the time and space to recover.

Support surrounds survivors during treatment. When it ends, not only is the support gone, everyone is celebrating and anxious for the survivor's life to begin again. Many survivors I've worked with share in the celebration but are soon discouraged that they still feel so bad. They may not want to burst everyone's bubble and joy of it being over (and at the time may not realize what's ahead). While not bursting bubbles can sound like a nice thing to do, it can actually create pressure to do more and thus set one back in terms of regaining energy and health. One survivor I coached struggled for months to tell her daughter she could not take care of her little ones. She suffered in silence, fatigued and depressed, hurting herself in the long run by not being able to be honest. Her depression was about not regaining her energy more quickly and getting back to the things she loved most. I imagine if her doctor had told her and her family that regaining strength and energy would take time, it may have helped create an open dialogue that it was okay to not be ready to take care of her grandchildren.

#77: Exercise is a non-negotiable component of recovery and may reduce your risk of recurrence.

As discussed in Chapters 5 and 6, exercise is medicine. Aerobic exercise increases blood flow, increases oxygen consumption, helps the body receive nutrients, removes waste, and helps maintain all vital systems that work together for our health. It has the ability to impact all of our body's systems at once (circulatory, digestive, endocrine, immune, lymphatic, muscular, nervous, respiratory, skeletal, etc.) and therefore help us heal, strengthen, and recover more quickly. When you think about post-surgery instructions, nurses want to get patients up and moving as soon as possible. Why? Because blood flow and oxygen to the tissues is increased and helps our body do what it needs to do to heal. Apply that to recovering from aggressive cancer treatment, and you can begin to see why it is so important! Our bodies were designed to move in order to work at an optimal level.

Aside from recovery, a life-long commitment to moving and exercise will work to keep other cancers and disease at bay. Regular exercise is also associated with a major reduction in risk of recurrence and death following a cancer diagnosis. The benefits are so powerful and numerous, it could truly be called a magic pill if you could swallow it!

Remember, what we are talking about when it comes to exercise being therapeutic is not just moving around the house, grocery shopping, or other busy activities. In fact, those activities can wear you out if you do too much. The type of exercise that will have the benefits listed in the following section is aerobic exercise that gets your heart rate up and pushes oxygen into the tissues, building endurance and energy storehouses each time you do it. The body responds to the new stress by adapting and getting stronger. The same is true for strength training. Strength training (or sometimes called resistance training), when done at an intensity or weight where you can only do 10 to 15 repetitions, will build strength and maintain or build lean muscle (see guidelines for both in Chapter 6: Optimal Well-Being During Treatment). We need muscle to keep our metabolism high, to prevent injury, to maintain strong bones, and to perform daily activities. Lack of muscle will eventually keep most people from taking care of themselves as they age.

Benefits of Exercise After Treatment

- Exercise improves healing and recovery, quality of life, sleep, self, confidence, energy, fatigue, depression, anxiety, energy, eases minor aches and pains, and strengthens the immune system.
- Research has shown that regular exercise may be associated with a reduced risk of recurrence and improved survival rates by as much as 40 to 50 percent over those who are not exercising regularly. The greatest benefit came when walking three to five hours per week at an average pace (2 to 2.9 mph).

- Survivors are at risk for developing other health conditions. Exercise reduces risk for heart disease, diabetes, stroke, obesity, and developing a second cancer. It reduces high blood pressure and cholesterol, circulates estrogen, builds muscle, strengthens bones, keeps the digestive system moving, and helps with weight loss and weight management. Exercise has been shown to reduce chronic inflammation, which may be an important factor in many chronic diseases, including cancer.

> For hormone-positive breast cancers, it's important to know that exercise reduces circulating estrogen (exercise increases SHBG, a sex hormone binding globulin, which picks up circulating estrogen). Also, our body fat produces estrogen (fat cells are a site of conversion of estrogen), so managing weight is an important goal.

Recommendations

Current recommendations are to follow national guidelines for cancer prevention that are listed in Chapter 6: Optimal Well-Being During Treatment. You should not expect to be back to pre-treatment levels of fitness immediately, and the time it takes varies from person to person. Fatigue may be cumulative with chemo and radiation, and you may experience more than you have had at any point after treatment ends. The long-term goal should be to meet the minimum guidelines and preferably double them over time for maximum benefit in lowering risk for disease, recurrence, and keeping weight under control.

When prioritizing tasks for the day, put exercise before everything, even if it is only 5 or 10 minutes when you first wake up. Build the minutes as weeks go by. Remember, being on your feet all day will not give you the same benefit. Focus on getting enough time in where you can safely work up to a brisk walk, forcing your heart and lungs to work harder. Be careful not to do too much too soon, and gradually progress your fitness level. If you are tired for the rest of the day after exercising, it is too much.

Exercise Tips

Because I know only one third of survivors follow the recommendations of exercise, and that when they are diagnosed, studies show that they decrease their physical activity by two hours a week (more if they are obese), I want to offer encouragement.

Of the women I've coached who never exercised regularly, most were able to successfully sustain a regular walking program when they started off with just five minutes a day. It was something they could easily commit to at first and by the end of three months could easily be doing 30 to 45 minutes in one workout. One client told me, "If you had told me I was going to be able to do this at the end of three months, or if you had said I *would be* doing 45 minutes, I would have probably quit. I wouldn't have believed it and would have been overwhelmed." For her and many others, it was committing to a baby step, writing it in on the calendar and schedule at a specific time, and feeling successful when that baby step was met. Before they knew it, they were adding more and more minutes to the schedule and feeling confident in their ability to sustain an exercise program.

Think of a tiny baby step you can take this week. Think about the exact time and place you will do it. Can you commit to five minutes of walking each day right after you wake up in the morning for the next five days? Whatever time or place it is, be specific with your commitment. For example: I will walk for five minutes around the building before getting in my car to go home from work on Monday, Wednesday, and Friday this week.

After you are able to walk at least 15 minutes at a brisk pace, consider interval training as a part of your workout to progress fitness more quickly. Interval training is where you alternate between "hard" and "easy" during the workout. The exact time for each part is not as important as thinking about working harder than normal for a short time and then slowing down to an easier pace to recover. Walking more briskly and super fast for 15 to 60 seconds and then walking moderately for 30 to 60 seconds (or longer for recovery) is an example of how this would be applied. Think about an athlete running sprints, but taking it down to a more comfortable level. Interval training can be done while riding a bike, walking, running, being on an elliptical trainer or treadmill. The intensity portion (when you are working harder) builds fitness levels more quickly than progressing at the same pace for the entire exercise session.

#78: Each time you eat or drink, you have an opportunity to strengthen and heal your body or weaken it.

Food is our fuel. Without it, we perish. The choices we make can support healing, overall health, a healthy weight, and a stronger immune system, or they can take away from it. Each time we eat, we have an opportunity to help our bodies be at an optimal working level. The fuel we put in our bodies can be super octane or low grade.

The information around nutrition is vast, and the best I can do in this small space is to encourage survivors to learn how to eat healthy, share a few key points, some guidelines, and offer the best resources for learning. A certified health or wellness coach can also help you follow through with the guidelines and recommendations to figure out the best way to incorporate healthy eating habits within the framework of *your* daily life.

What we know for sure is that our bodies function better when they are supported with a variety of brightly colored fruits and vegetables, less saturated fat, whole grains, and healthy lean proteins. Most Americans get enough protein in their diet, but because it rebuilds and repairs damaged tissue, you want to make sure you are getting enough (check with dietitian or go to www.choosemyplate.gov).

In general, supplements are not recommended, and research suggests aside from not really doing much for us, they may actually cause harm. Dietitians recommend that nutrients come from the foods we eat versus pill form. Sometimes supplements are recommended, such as Calcium and Vitamin D, but it's important to talk to your doctor or registered dietitian about what is right for you. Research has shown that cancer survivors take more supplements and may be more vulnerable to buying products or supplements that lack evidence of benefit and safety, at a significant financial cost. Further, taking too much of a nutrient may inhibit other nutrients from being utilized appropriately and causing deficiencies.

In a study published in the *Journal of Clinical Oncology*, researchers found that survivors might be vulnerable to unsubstantiated claims of benefits from supplements. When researchers visited 34 health food stores asking about supplements for cancer survivors, they found that employees were:
- Giving advice with little or no training
- Giving advice that was misleading, wrong, or potentially harmful
- Discussing possible cures (with supplements)

They also said survivors, as with the general public, may believe that supplements are safe because they occur in nature. The authors said, "This study highlighted the vulnerability of patients with breast cancer to potentially misleading information from health food employees. Advice presented by health food employees was authoritative and could be misconstrued by patients as evidence-based, particularly when books are consulted or literature is provided on the products." My advice: Buyer beware.

The science around food and nutrition is growing in regards to learning what will have an impact on cancer, both positively and negatively. Inflammation has been linked to cancer and other disease processes, for example. The foods we choose may serve to reduce inflammation or increase it. Taking anti-inflammatory medications on a regular basis can be risky to our stomachs and intestinal health, so choosing healthy foods that will minimize or reduce inflammation may be helpful. These foods are not weird, exotic concoctions, but a variety of healthy foods we should all have in our diets. Sugar, white flour, processed foods, and other junk food may increase inflammation (and may contribute to obesity). In the book *Anticancer*, Servan-Schreiber goes into great detail around these concepts. They are currently being studied in clinical trials at M.D. Anderson Cancer Center, in Houston.

Cancer survivors should follow national guidelines for cancer prevention. In other words, we should follow healthy eating patterns just like everyone, to reduce our risk for other cancers, recurrence, and other diseases. Several major organizations have guidelines for us to follow.

American Cancer Society Recommendations

- Eat a balanced diet, rich in fruits and vegetables.
- Lower fat intake.
- Avoid or limit intake of alcoholic beverages.
- Manage weight by limiting calories.
- Get active. Exercise vigorously at least five times a week for 50 to 60 minutes.

American Institute of Cancer Research Recommendations (www.AICR.org)

- Be as lean as possible without becoming underweight.
- Be physically active for at least 30 minutes every day.
- Avoid sugary drinks. Limit consumption of energy-dense foods.
- Eat more of a variety of vegetables, fruits, whole grains, and legumes such as beans.
- Limit consumption of red meats (such as beef, pork, and lamb), and avoid processed meats.
- If consumed at all, limit alcoholic drinks to two for men and one for women per day.
- Limit consumption of salty foods and foods processed with salt (sodium).
- Don't use supplements to protect against cancer.

- It is best for mothers to breastfeed exclusively for up to six months and then add other liquids and foods.
- After treatment, cancer survivors should follow the recommendations for cancer prevention.

USDA Dietary Guidelines for Americans, 2010 (www.choosemyplate.org)

The overall focus for the new guidelines is on balancing calories with physical activity, consuming more healthy foods like vegetables, fruits, whole grains, fat-free and low-fat dairy products, and seafood, and consuming less sodium, saturated and trans fats, added sugars, and refined grains.

- Enjoy your food, but eat less.
- Avoid oversized portions.
- Make half your plate fruits and vegetables (www.fruitsandveggiesmatter.gov).
- Switch to fat-free or low-fat (1%) milk.
- Compare sodium in foods like soup, bread, and frozen meals, and choose the foods with lower numbers.
- Drink water instead of sugary drinks.

Foods and Food Components to Reduce

- Reduce daily sodium intake to less than 2,300 milligrams (mg), and further reduce intake to 1,500 mg (equivalent to 3/4 teaspoon salt per day) among persons who are 51 and older and those of any age who are African American or have hypertension, diabetes, or chronic kidney disease. The 1,500 mg recommendation applies to about half of the U.S. population, including children, and the majority of adults.
- Consume less than 10 percent of calories from saturated fatty acids by replacing them with monounsaturated and polyunsaturated fatty acids.
- Consume less than 300 mg per day of dietary cholesterol.
- Keep trans fatty acid consumption as low as possible by limiting foods that contain synthetic sources of trans fats, such as partially hydrogenated oils, and by limiting other solid fats.
- Reduce the intake of calories from solid fats (things like shortening that are solid at room temperature) and added sugars.
- Limit the consumption of foods that contain refined grains, especially refined grain foods that contain solid fats, added sugars, and sodium.
- If alcohol is consumed, it should be consumed in moderation—up to one drink per day for women and two drinks per day for men—and only by adults of legal drinking age.

Foods and Nutrients to Increase

Individuals should meet the following recommendations as part of a healthy eating pattern while staying within their calorie needs:

- Increase vegetable and fruit intake.
- Eat a variety of vegetables, especially dark green and red and orange vegetables and beans and peas.
- Consume at least half of all grains as whole grains. Increase whole-grain intake by replacing refined grains with whole grains.
- Increase intake of fat-free or low-fat milk and milk products, such as milk, yogurt, cheese, or fortified soy beverages.
- Choose a variety of protein foods, which include seafood, lean meat and poultry, eggs, beans and peas, soy products, and unsalted nuts and seeds.
- Increase the amount and variety of seafood consumed by choosing seafood in place of some meat and poultry.
- Replace protein foods that are higher in solid fats with choices that are lower in solid fats and calories and/or are sources of oils.
- Use oils to replace solid fats where possible.
- Choose foods that provide more potassium, dietary fiber, calcium, and vitamin D, which are nutrients of concern in American diets. These foods include vegetables, fruits, whole grains, and milk products.

Other Diet-Related Concerns for Survivors

Soy and Flaxseed Recommendations

Soy and flaxseed have been studied in relationship to their ability to act on breast cancer cells. Under certain conditions, soy and flaxseed can mimic the actions of hormones, like estrogen, while other times they may counteract them. Research is ongoing, so stay updated by going to sites like the American Institute of Cancer Research (AICR). Always check with your doctor before making special modifications to your diet such as these.

Some scientists believe that soy may have anti-cancer effects, but there's limited evidence in U.S. populations that it might offer special protection. Asian women who have eaten soy since adolescence appear to have a lower incidence of breast cancer, but that doesn't necessarily mean it would be true for American women who start eating it in adulthood. The most current thinking in regards to soy is that one or two servings of soy food products per day (like soy nuts, tofu or edamame) are now considered relatively safe for survivors, but soy supplements are not. The AICR says that, as a precaution, women receiving anti-estrogen treatments (such as tamoxifen) should minimize soy foods and avoid isoflavone supplements.

Flaxseed appears to be safe as an omega-3 fat for breast cancer survivors, but research is also limited in human studies in regards to breast cancer risk/benefits. In animal studies, it did appear to decrease growth of estrogen positive/negative breast cancers. In a small human study, 5 to 30 grams per day (1 to 4 T ground flaxseed—not flaxseed oil that may not carry the effective properties), altered estrogen metabolism in a way that showed a protective effect. Research to confirm that it is protective is limited, but it may be helpful in small amounts. If you want to consume it, make sure to discuss with your doctor as it can interfere with some medications.

Green Tea

In the laboratory (not in humans), green tea has been shown to slow or stop the development of breast cancer cells. But, in AICR's expert report, Food, Nutrition, Physical Activity, and the Prevention of Cancer: A Global Perspective, scientists were unable to make recommendations about consumption due to a lack of evidence. The National Cancer Institute states that after 50 studies published around tea consumption and cancer risk since 2006, results were inconclusive as to the benefits. Though most experts believe it is safe when consumed moderately, and may be even be potentially helpful, they did not have the science to back a recommendation. Research can be complicated when it comes to nutritional factors. People may respond differently due to their genetic makeup or other lifestyle factors that may also contribute to risk.

It is important to know that very high amounts of green tea components, such as in supplements, have been shown to impact drugs that affect blood clotting, like aspirin. Green tea has strong binding properties (polyphenols) that may impact medications you are taking. Green tea does have caffeine, so know it can also impact sleep, if you don't get the decaffeinated form. More controlled and randomized studies on humans are currently in the works, so stay tuned.

More About Managing Weight With Nutrition and Exercise

Weight loss is a math calculation: calories in versus calories out. Just 100 calories more than your body needs in a day will add up to 10 pounds gained in one year. Likewise, walking about a mile a day (roughly equivalent to 100 calories) will result in a loss of 10 pounds in one year, if all other factors remain the same.

It is very possible to gain weight even when eating a diet full of healthy foods! Legumes, or beans, for example, can pack a wallop of calories if portion sizes are too large. Calories still matter. A healthy weight is extremely important for breast cancer survivors, reducing our risk for recurrence, disease, and other cancers. So eat healthy, but watch the calories as well.

Remember that weight didn't get on you overnight, so take the same slow and steady approach, but in the reverse. Focus on healthy habits: staying active, exercising, and eating more fruits and vegetables (while minimizing high-calorie foods). Write down what you eat (to see what the reality is, even if for just a few days), and use a pedometer to track your activity levels. Weight loss will follow. It's what you do consistently and for the long haul that matters. As we age, we have to eat less, and actively seek to exercise and move our bodies more. As we age, we lose muscle, and that impacts the calories we burn at rest. We have to do everything we can to keep the balance where it needs to be. The most important factors for weight management are to do strength training to maintain muscle (that helps your calorie burning potential at rest), eat foods high in nutrients but low in calories, such as fruits and vegetables and lean proteins, and get plenty of physical activity and exercise (wear a pedometer, shooting for 10,000 steps a day). All of that will tip the calorie balance in your favor.

Mindset Matters

I know personally how difficult weight management can be and understand the frustration of feeling like you are doing everything you can, and the weight won't budge. It is more challenging as we age, but it is possible.

In listening to women about their experience of treatment for breast cancer and understanding what it was like for myself, gaining weight adds insult to injury. We all have been through so much. Struggling to lose it is just one more challenge and frustration.

One woman summed her feelings up in an online discussion, by talking about all she had been through and did not want to feel guilty about gaining weight:

> "I am an 18-month breast cancer survivor. With so many 'factors' alluding to breast cancer and breast cancer recurrence, how can we know what is or isn't something to take seriously? I am in fairly good shape, but overweight—after a bilateral, chemo, and hysterectomy over a 10-month span felt that I did all I can do to stay healthy. All of that, combined with being thrown into menopause during the process, has contributed to weight gain. Now, I feel guilty for gaining weight! I agree that there are many things we have to do to take care of ourselves, but I don't want to feel guilty about being heavier now than I was before."

Another responds:

> "I did not have to do the chemo or radiation treatments, but with five surgeries and still in the reconstruction phase, it's been a challenge to stay healthy, mentally, physically and then to have the energy to focus on eating healthy, which you would think after cancer it would be a priority. I feel down often about my weight as I do not fit any clothes, and I am not working, so it's not like I can just go out shopping to buy news clothes to feel better!"

I understand and empathize with these common feelings of frustration. We have been dealt a blow to our bodies that can be maddening at times. We can't change that, but what we can do is take control of what we can. Yes, it stinks. The question then becomes, now what? Do I want to stay in this place? Staying stuck in this frustration will only lead us in a downward spiral of health, where taking action will give us hope.

Changing focus and motivation from "weight loss" to doing the things that will make you feel better, live longer, and have more energy can be more empowering. For example, when I exercise, I have less aches and pains and am less fatigued. I have more energy and simply feel better. When I eat healthier, I feel better and have more energy. Women I coach often say they want to lose weight because they want to be able to play with their grandchildren or do some other fun activities they have been unable to do. Others are motivated by the fact that healthy weight and exercising has been shown to reduce risk for recurrence. Whatever it is, find what motivates you, and focus on that vision of well-being.

Specific Resources for Nutrition

- American Institute for Cancer Research (www.AICR.org): Website to learn the latest research and recommendations related to cancer and lifestyle
- Cancer Dietitian (www.cancerdietitian.com): A cancer dietitian (CSO) covers topics that survivors often ask about.
- USDA (www.choosemyplate.gov): Learn more details of a healthy eating plan
- *Anticancer, A New Way of Life* by David Servan-Schreiber. Book mentioned in Chapter 6: Optimal Well-Being During Treatment.

#79: A focused wellness plan will help you recover in the optimal amount of time possible.

A focused plan is critical to regain health, energy, and vitality from the toll that cancer treatment takes on the body. With no plan, it will take much longer, and in some cases health can continue into a downward spiral. You can come up with your own plan or work with a professional to help you develop one.

A certified health or wellness coach, with a background in health and fitness, can help with an overall plan to improve health and well-being that is comprehensive, covering all parts of your life, and specifically, outlining action steps. Some background or training in working with cancer survivors is especially helpful. Most of the time, the service is delivered by phone, so there are no geographical boundaries. It is private, and convenient for most people.

A wellness coach works with individuals to think about what changes they want to make, what matters most to them, and plan the best way to move forward. As mentioned in Chapter 6, my Healthy and Fit After Cancer program (wellness coaching for cancer survivors) was the subject of research published in late 2009 and was shown to reduce anxiety, depression, and body weight, and increase physical activity, fruit and vegetable consumption, and overall quality of life for survivors, both in the short and long term. As a co-investigator on the study and a coach, I believe that some of the reasons wellness coaching was successful are as follows:

- It was comprehensive in scope, with all parts of a person's life included in the conversation.
- Participants had a chance to be still and *think* about what mattered, find their specific motivation for change, and think about what they wanted to do, formulating a step-by-step action plan.
- The process built confidence in their ability to take action and sustain the positive changes.
- The professional background and expertise of the coach in exercise and lifestyle change (knowledge of applicable national guidelines) may have been helpful for guidance and support when needed.
- The partnership between client and coach was built on trust, rapport, empathy, and positive regard for one another in a judgment-free zone.
- Participants determined the agenda and scope of their program.

Go to www.HealthyandFitAfterCancer.com for more information about wellness coaching for cancer survivors.

SELF-COACHING TIPS IN DEVELOPING A PLAN

Know where you want to go. Having a plan is a first step to getting there. Write down what you want. Create a vision board or a vision statement about what your life will look like when you have the optimal health and well-being you want. Don't forget to include all parts of your life that contribute to your well-being. Think about the things that make you thrive and flourish, and include them in your plan.

What are the behaviors you need to be doing on a regular basis to get you to that vision? For example, if you want to lose weight, what behaviors do you want/need to be doing consistently? Exercising 30 to 45 minutes, five days a week? Eating at least 5 to 10 servings of fruits and vegetables every day? Taking 10,000 steps each day? Think of the behaviors, set a goal, and then take baby steps to reach them.

Example Plans

Fitness

- Three-month goal: I will walk 30 minutes 5 days a week.
- First week goal: I will walk five minutes on Monday, Wednesday, and Friday morning at 7 a.m. before having my coffee.

Nutrition

- Three-month goal: I will eat at least five fruits and vegetables, six out of seven days a week.
- First week goal: I will bring an apple to work for my afternoon snack on Tuesday and Thursday.

Sleep

- Three-month goal: I will sleep at least seven hours each night.
- First week goal: I will call and make an appointment on Monday morning to talk to my doctor about my sleep issues.

OTHER SPECIALIZED SERVICES THAT CAN SUPPORT YOUR OVERALL WELLNESS AND WELLNESS PLAN

As mentioned in Chapter 6: Optimal Well-Being During Treatment, the list of support professionals and programs may or may not be covered by insurance or supported by grants. After treatment the focus will be slightly different but many of the professionals will be the same.

Survivorship programs are often found in cancer centers and other non-profit support organizations that assist survivors in learning how to transition from treatment to life after treatment—from psycho-social support (counseling/support) to exercise recovery programs.

Cancer rehabilitation programs are usually offered in medically based fitness centers or through a physical therapy department/clinic, and can offer the first step to regain strength and function.

Integrative medicine programs offer many mind-body healing programs that can be helpful such as yoga, stress-reduction classes, acupuncture, massage, as well as other services listed here.

Physical therapy (PT) or occupational therapy (OT) professionals work closely with cancer centers to provide services to cancer survivors and help them regain daily functioning. Specific services with PTs and OTs are usually covered by insurance.

Personal trainers or fitness specialists are invaluable in having supervision of a trained exercise professional to progress your fitness safely. Look for a trainer who has the ACSM/ACS cancer and exercise certification or specialized training in order to help you. All trainers are not trained equally.

Dietitians with a board certification in oncology as well as other registered and licensed dietitians can answer questions you may have about nutrition moving forward.

Social workers/counselors can help you move through the transition after treatment and support you with your emotional well-being.

Sexual health professionals can provide specific guidance to challenges above and beyond what a gynecologist or oncology professional may provide.

Health or wellness coaches with expertise in exercise, nutrition, and weight management experience, as mentioned above, can help you facilitate changes and optimize hope, health, and overall well-being.

These professionals with professional coach training are an added bonus (like a dietitian or personal trainer), as they not only can share expert information, they can help you apply and facilitate the information within the context of your life.

#80: Hormone-replacement therapy is not a safe option for dealing with hot flashes.

Survivors should not take hormone replacement therapy (HRT) if they have hormone sensitive breast cancer (estrogen- or progesterone-positive breast cancer) because estrogen may assist breast cancer cells to grow and spread. Some doctors may also recommend that women with hormone-negative cancers avoid HRT.

No scientific data is available to support the claim that bio-identical hormones are any safer, and they carry the same risks as hormones that are prescribed. All bio-identical hormones are synthetically created, like other HRT. Bio-identical hormones are made in a pharmacy and have not undergone strict scientific study; therefore, there is no guarantee of safety, purity, or efficacy.

Soy supplements are not safe to use, and very few herbal remedies have proven to be effective. Be cautious of any product or supplement that mimics estrogen. Prescription drugs such as anti-depressants have been used effectively for some women in reducing hot flashes.

Many women in our culture have assumed that we must take HRT in order to "get through" menopause. Though it can be extremely challenging to go through immediate menopause (because of chemotherapy or hysterectomy), it is possible to manage it. This type of menopause can be more severe than regular menopause that normally progresses over 5 to 10 years.

A combination of strategies can be helpful, such as healthy lifestyle behaviors like exercise. One particular study showed that women who exercise have half the hot flashes of those that are sedentary. Deep breathing has been shown to reduce hot flashes by 40 percent (six to eight breaths per minute) when done at least two times per day.

I experienced a sudden and severe menopause that caused me to have hot flashes I was sure could power a small town. I kept a small battery operated fan around at all times, had an oscillating fan by my bed to turn on me when I woke with a flash (still do), wore light cotton night clothing, and during the day dressed light or in layers. I used deep breathing to bring on a relaxation response when I felt one coming on and drank cold water if it was nearby. Was it easy? No. Sometimes, I think I had them every other minute. Was it comfortable? Heavens no. But there are worse things in life to have to deal with.

For me, the common triggers of anxiety, stress, caffeine (chocolate, tea, coffee), spicy foods, and warmer than comfortable temperatures always brought them on, so I did my best to minimize them.

#81: Alcohol may be associated with risk of recurrence.

Researchers followed early stage breast cancer survivors for eight years and found that three to four drinks per week was associated with a 30 percent increased risk of recurrence for survivors who were postmenopausal and overweight or obese. Interestingly, women who were of a normal body weight or BMI did not show an increased risk of recurrence in this study.

#82: Annual breast screenings are still important.

After a bout with breast cancer, survivors don't always understand the need to continue their annual mammograms. In fact, many put it off. What all survivors need to know is that there is a small chance of having another "primary" cancer in the other breast (not a recurrence, but a new cancer).

It's important to discuss screening on the affected breast as well, because even though breast tissue may have been removed in a mastectomy, cells can sometimes still remain in the breast or under the arm. There is always a small chance that a second primary or recurrence can occur in the affected breast when there was no mastectomy and a lumpectomy was performed. Paying attention to changes, knowing your body, and using your intuition is still important for early detection. Refer to Chapter 2: Early Detection for more information.

I know of one woman who had her cancer return underneath her implant. By the time it was caught, it was too late, and she passed away within a few months. I share that not to scare women, but to emphasize that we are no different than others in detecting problems early.

Because you are at high risk, insurance may pay for you to have an annual MRI or other imaging in addition to mammography. Talk to your doctor about the best screening for your situation. All regular health screenings continue to be important, regardless of cancer status.

#83: Sexual health is affected in nearly all survivors and is an important part of our well-being, so don't give up.

According to the American Cancer Society, an estimated 90 percent of survivors report their sexuality being affected in some way. Sadly, less than a third talk to their providers about the change. Because it is a topic that is hard or embarrassing to talk about, many women suffer in silence. Privately, survivors discuss the frustration of yet one more devastating side effect and may exchange ideas with a close friend. But often, they give up, resigning themselves to the loss, not knowing help is available.

In an Australian study of 1,600 women under age 70, 70 percent had sexual problems within two years after their diagnosis, even though they had a good and satisfying sex lives beforehand. Almost half of the women felt different about their body image, yet only 12 percent said their partners were unhappy about their appearance. And in spite of the challenges, two thirds of the women *did* want to increase their sexual desire. Researchers found that women taking drugs that blocked estrogen and those who received chemotherapy had more difficulties than those who did not.

Between fatigue, physical changes from surgery, radiation, or chemo (loss of hair, breast surgery, etc.) and experiencing a life-threatening illness, it is no surprise why a woman might not feel like being physically intimate. However, the challenge is much more than the difficulty of treatment. Many of the treatments for breast cancer reduce or block estrogen levels and which may lead to vaginal dryness, atrophy of tissues, and loss of libido or desire. Intercourse can become painful, which further compounds the problem of lowered desire. Who wants to do something that is painful?

One of the most exciting parts of writing this book, for me, is being able to report the following great news around this topic. There is hope! Medical specialists have dedicated their lives to helping women (and men) who have experienced health changes that impact their sexuality. A satisfying sex life is possible and an important part of our overall health and well-being.

What You Can Do

Many levels of solutions are available, starting with the most simple to more specialized assistance from experts in the field of sexual health:

- First, don't give up on sex prematurely. It is a special bond between two people in love that is worth striving to keep! Even if you don't have a partner and think you don't care if you ever have sex again, there are reasons to maintain the health of these parts of our body. Avoiding infections and maintaining healthy tissues for future relationships, should you change your mind, are among a few. As we've learned, we can't predict the future!

- Learn more about the changes that are taking place so you can be proactive. The low estrogen state of tissues can cause thinning, burning, itching, and dryness and make us more susceptible to vaginal infections, as well as recurrent urinary tract infections (UTIs). The goal is to restore moisture, elasticity, natural pH, and comfort to the tissues.
- Know the difference between vaginal moisturizers and lubricants, and use them both. Use moisturizers for adding moisture back to vaginal walls, internally. Think of using them in the same light as using facial moisturizers. Lubricants are for comfort during sexual activity and are always used externally.
- Lubricants are best when they are water- or silicone-based, liquid or gel. Oil-based products can harbor bacteria, get into the urethra, and contribute to urinary tract or bladder infections. Avoid glycerin, warming, icing, cooling, or scented gels, as they can cause irritation. Silicone and glycerin in lubricants can contribute to yeast infections, so if you are prone to them, use water-based products only. Lubricants should be applied to you and your partner. In a presentation discussing sexuality for Living Beyond Breast Cancer, Dr. Spadt said her patients liked the following lubricants:
    - ✓ *Astroglide Organic, Wet Silk* (silicone product), *Slippery Stuff* (some only found online)
    - ✓ The very favorite: *Good Clean Love's Almost Naked Organic Personal Lubricant*
- Moisturizers work to restore moisture and elasticity to the vagina, improving the balance of intracellular fluids and increasing water to the cells. They should be used regularly and can be used two to three times per week or more, whether having sex or not.
    - ✓ Dr. Spadt's patients preferred the following products: *Me Again, Good Clean Love, KY-Liquid Beads*. Others she referred to were: Replens
    - ✓ The very favorite of patients: *Me Again Vaginal Moisturizer*
- Have intercourse or use vaginal dilators regularly to minimize atrophy or shrinking of the vaginal tissue. Vaginal dilators can be prescribed and are made of materials like glass, silicone, or plastic. Be careful about using materials that might harbor bacteria (soft). Physical therapists who specialize in women's health can be helpful if you need assistance in this area.
- Do Kegel exercises before sex. When intercourse has had a history of being painful, muscles will tense up in anticipation. Working these muscles right before intercourse will keep them from tensing up by fatiguing them and allowing an easier experience.
- Communicate your needs and desire to continue or improve your sex life with your partner. They need to know that you care and want it to continue. Our relationships change as we age, with or without cancer. Sex is not the same at 20 as it is at 40 as it is at 70, but it can be an opportunity to deepen your relationship, improve intimacy, and have an even better sex life than before.

- Most experts will tell us that the most important organ involved in sexual activity is our mind: "Sex happens mostly between our ears." Do what you can to create the mindset and intention for a positive outcome. Focus on the love you have with your partner and being close to them. Buy lingerie that feels sensuous to you and that covers areas you might be shy or uncomfortable about. Read romantic or erotic materials (therapists call it bibliotherapy) two to three times a week.

- Seek help from a sex therapist if these simpler strategies are not working. Experts trained in the field can help you, just as in any other health issue. Know that a comfortable and enjoyable sex life is possible.

Specific Resources

- The American Physical Therapy Association or APTA (www.apta.org) is a resource for finding a therapist who can help you with physical issues related to sexual health in women (and are usually female). Look under "Find a therapist," then specify "Women's Health" and look for specialties such as dyspeurenia (pain during intercourse), or related topics to the pelvic floor by each therapist's specialization. Local therapists may be able to refer you to a colleague if they are not the right fit.

- Books on this topic are starting to become more numerous, so keep an eye out for them. I highly recommend *100 Questions & Answers About Breast Cancer Sensuality, Sexuality, and Intimacy* by Drs. Michael Krychman, MD, Susan Kellogg Spadt, PhD, DRNP, and Sandra Finestone, PsyD.

- The Center for Intimacy After Cancer Therapy (renewintimacy.org/counseling.aspx) is a non-profit that can provide counseling by phone for individuals or couples.

- Go to the Sexual Health Network (www.aasect.org) to find a nationally certified sex therapist.

#84: Your mindset matters.

Learning to flourish and reach optimal health and well-being is more than just doing some of the things mentioned above. Martin Seligman, the father of positive psychology, believes there are five basic areas that contribute to well-being and our ability to flourish: positive emotion, engagement, positive relationships, meaning, and achievement.

As human beings, we have to work to build positive emotions, but that doesn't mean being a Pollyanna with a smile on our face all the time. It's about increasing positive emotions like joy, gratitude, serenity, interest, hope, pride, amusement, inspiration, awe, and love.

Working diligently to balance the negative thoughts and emotions that come our way—with a 3:1 positive to negative ratio—has been shown to increase our ability to flourish or thrive. Positive emotions help us develop closer connections with others, build resilience and optimism, as well as be less depressed and more satisfied with life.

Only 10 percent of our happiness is attributed to our life's circumstances, 50 percent is basically a set point/genetic and we can't really change it, but the remaining 40 percent is under our control. We can cultivate optimism and happiness for ourselves.

- Make it a daily practice to grow positive emotions and create a 3:1 ratio. Barbara Fredrickson's book *Positivity* explains the science behind that ratio and gives fabulous exercises for building our positivity ratio.
- Focus on what is going well and is working, instead of what is not working or going well. What you focus on will grow.
- Focus on what you have control of, instead of what you don't.

Enjoy some GRASS, an acronym I came up with to remember what you can do to flourish. Think about walking barefoot in a soft bed of green grass to bring a positive association and remember the acronym.

- *Give back:* Performing acts of kindness is highly correlated with happiness, improves self-image and a sense of community. Volunteering has been shown to lifts spirits no matter how busy or how badly people felt beforehand. They always felt better when they volunteered.

  A colleague of mine with muscular dystrophy only has two hours every day that she can function. She had a revelation that even while she was lying in bed she could make a difference. She said she could send compassionate loving thoughts and prayer to specific people and the world!
- *Relationships:* People with strong ties to friends and family and a commitment to spending time with them have the highest levels of happiness and the fewest signs of depression. You don't have to have large numbers of friends—just a few good friends that you stay engaged with!

- ***Appreciation:*** Having gratitude and appreciation for anything in any given moment is sure to take you out of the past and future, landing you right in the present to savor. Gratitude can shift your mood like nothing else. When researchers had people write down three things they appreciated or were grateful for each night for one week (and what role they might have played in that), they were happier than a control group six months later. Writing a letter of gratitude and delivering it to someone in person (not a relative) was also shown to significantly improve happiness for at least one month.

- ***Strengths:*** Understanding and building on personal strengths has been shown to improve well-being. Utilizing personal strengths in a new way every day for at least a week was shown to improve and sustain happiness over a control group six months later. Researchers studied cultures around the world and found shared character strengths and virtues common to all human beings. To find your top strengths, a free assessment is available at www.authentichappiness.org. Scroll down and find the VIA Signature Strengths assessment. You will receive a list of your top character strengths, and you can then plan to use them daily. If creativity is one of your strengths, for example, you would find activities that utilize and engage your creative side. Utilizing your strengths will also keep you highly engaged in your life, an important part of the "thriving" formula.

- ***Savor:*** Taking time to savor the past, present, and future can build positive emotions and reduce worry or anxiety.

  ✓ Past: Reflect and reminisce about past experiences. Positive reminiscence, or building positive memories around times that may not have been so great, can reduce anxiety in the present. Thinking about lessons learned, positive experiences amidst the hard time, and people who were there to support you can allow you to draw strength from the memory. Forgiveness is also a powerful action that allows us to let go of pain and move forward.

  ✓ Present: Savoring the present moment can prolong an enjoyable moment, like a vaccination, making it last longer. Savoring the present can take you away from worry about the future or thoughts about the past, where most anxiety comes from.

  ✓ Future: Positive anticipation of the future is about hope. Whether it is planning for 10 minutes from now or 10 years, goals and plans give rise to hope. Enjoy dreaming and planning!

Chapter References

The American Institute of Cancer Research
www.aicr.org.

The Cancer Support Community
www.csc.BreastCancerRegistry.org.

Holmes, M., Chen, W.D.F., Kroenke, C., & Colditz, G. (2005). Physical activity and survival after breast cancer diagnosis. *JAMA*. 293(20): 2479–2486.

Irwin, M.L., Crumley, D., McTiernan, A., et al (2003). Physical activity levels before and after a diagnosis of breast carcinoma: the Health, Eating, Activity, and Lifestyle (HEAL) study. *Cancer*. 97: 1746–1757.

Irwin, M.L., McTiernan, A., Bernstein, L., et al (2004). Physical activity levels among breast cancer survivors. *Med Sci Sports Exerc*. 36: 1484–1491

Irwin, M.L., Smith, A.W., McTiernan, A., et al (2008). Influence of pre- and postdiagnosis physical activity on mortality in breast cancer survivors: the health, eating, activity, and lifestyle study. *J Clin Oncol*. 26: 3958–3964.

Kwan, M.L., et al (2010). Alcohol consumption and breast cancer recurrence and survival among women with early-stage breast cancer: the life after cancer epidemiology study. *Journal of Clinical Oncology*. Oct 10, 28(29): 4410–4416.

Larsson, S.C., Akesson, A., Bergkvist, L., & Wolk, A. (2010). Multivitamin use and breast cancer incidence in a prospective cohort of Swedish women. *Am J Clin Nutr*. May, 91(5): 1268–1272.

Miller, P., Demark-Wahnefried, W., Snyder, D., Sloane, R., Morey, M., Cohen, H., Kranz, S., Mitchell, D., & Hartman, T. (2008) Dietary supplement use among elderly, long-term cancer survivors. *J Cancer Surviv*. Sept., 2(3): 138–148.

Mills, E., Ernst, E., Singh, R., Ross, C., & Wilson, K. (2003). Health food store recommendations: implications for breast cancer patients. *Breast Cancer Res*. 5(6): R170–174.

Pierce, J.P., Natarajan, L., Caan, B.J., Parker, B.A., Greenberg, E.R., Flatt, S.W., et al (2007). Influence of a diet very high in vegetables, fruit, and fiber and low in fat on prognosis following treatment for breast cancer: The Women's Healthy Eating and Living (WHEL) randomized trial. *JAMA*. July, 298(3): 289–298.

Rock, C.L., Flatt, S.W., Natarajan, L., Thomson, C.A., Bardwell, W.A., Newman, V.A., et al (2005). Plasma carotenoids and recurrence-free survival in women with a history of breast cancer. *Journal of Clinical Oncology*. Sept., 23(27): 6631–6638.

Schmitz, K.H., Courneya, K.S., Matthews, C., Demark-Wahnefried, W., Galvao, D.A., Pinto, B.M., Irwin, M.L., Wolin, K.Y., Segal, R.J., Lucia, A., Schneider, C.M., & von Gruenigen, V.E. (2010). ACSM Roundtable on exercise for cancer survivors. *Medicine & Science in Sports & Exercise*. 42(7): 1409–1426.

Schmitz, K.H. et al (2009). Weight lifting in women with breast-cancer–related lymphedema. *New England Journal of Medicine*. 361: 664–673.

8

Giving, Receiving, and Seeking Support

Knowing how to support others going through a rough time is something we are not necessarily born knowing how to do, but it is something we can learn. Reading this book is the first step to understanding the experience with empathy. The more you know, the more you can understand about how to help.

I don't pretend to have all the answers, but I know how it feels when someone says or does something that is helpful! Support comes in many forms, from a simple acknowledgment and kind word to enormous gestures, to connecting with others going through the same experience.

The outpouring of kindness from humanity during a difficult time, including that from strangers, is a beautiful thing. As in the words from Gilda Radner mentioned in Chapter 6: Optimal Well-Being During Treatment, everyone should get to feel the upside of cancer (one of which is the support and kindness), but of course, there is a huge downside.

And it's important to say that the "patient" experiencing treatment is not the only survivor. As you'll see in Chapter 9: Survivorship, the definition includes those who love and care for them. It is a different experience to be a co-survivor, one that can often lead to feelings of helplessness and frustration. We want the best for our loved ones, and yet we are not in control of their choices or the outcome. Loving someone who is going through cancer treatment means you don't want to see them suffer or go through a challenging time, but you also want them to live. You can help your loved one in many ways detailed in this chapter. But you can also help them by taking care of yourself, just as you would ask of them, so you can be your best for them, following many of the items discussed in Chapters 6 and 7.

We can do or say many different things to support each other throughout the survivorship journey. Much of what is shared in this chapter can be applied to other diseases and difficult situations where a friend or loved one is facing a challenge.

People deal with cancer in their own way. Some people want lots of information, while others let a caregiver take the lead, unable to face the details. Some people are private and don't want to talk or let people know they have cancer; others will tell just a few, while others will be an open book. Sometimes, even the most open person wants to just be alone, or a mix of both at times.

Sometimes, people want to be alone to sort out what they are feeling and not share the whole process with others as they are evolving through it, protecting those around from the ups and downs and worrying those close. With energy levels at an all-time low, even the smallest of activities can be an energy drain. Other times, being with a friend who is able to be a calming presence gives energy.

Friends or family may also deal with cancer in their own way. Survivors may find that the people they thought would be there in their greatest moment of need back away, while others they never imagined step in for the duration. It is disconcerting, but we can't control how others react.

Still, there are those people who are living with cancer and its treatment for the rest of their lives (Stage IV). Their way of dealing with the situation will be as individual as we all are as human beings. I have known many people to live as fully and inspirationally as any human being for years, with an attitude of "I am living *with*, not dying *from* cancer." "We are all terminal," as my friend Suzanne Lindley says. When we have a diagnosis of cancer, it just makes us all aware of that fact.

In the spirit of illustrating the very real thoughts and emotions around support and around a new diagnosis and treatment, I am sharing the following pieces from emails sent at the beginning of treatment and after (almost a year later) to friends and family. It illustrates the wide variety of emotions a diagnosis brings and how much even the smallest gestures of support can mean.

> "SOOOOO... How am I doing? I am very, very tired and worn out, but aside from that, the answer varies minute to minute. It's still hard to believe that this 'healthy' body has cancer. I am an emotional roller coaster. I am the same strong Pam everyone sees on the outside, getting information, being assertive, going about the business of being proactive and getting the job done of dealing with the big C ... On the other hand, you might find me crying at any point during the day, or laughing, or thanking God for the blessings in my life, or feeling like it's too much. One of the hardest things for me is having people do for me... and what the interruption means to my family—what a pain! I am

working on accepting this part. As a fellow coach said, 'Think of letting people help you as your gift to them...because people want to help.' That's tough!"

After nearly a year of treatment, these words summarize the value of reaching out, in an email written to those who supported me:

"Thank you for all of the kind words you all had for me. Everyone contributed in their own way ... it's amazing how just a few heartfelt expressions coming from EVERY ONE of you made me feel so cared for and loved during this difficult time. Thank you for the gifts of being who you are."

So no matter how large or small a gesture, they all represent kindness, love, and support to someone in the throes of cancer treatment and recovery.

#85: Having compassion for oneself will make the journey easier.

If your compassion does not include yourself, it is incomplete.
—Jack Kornfield

Most of us are able to show compassion, love, and empathy for others, but when it comes to giving it to ourselves, we fall short. If there is any time in your life to give yourself a break and show compassion for yourself, it is now, whether a patient, partner, family member, or friend. They say you can't give what you don't have.

It's the kind of compassion you might give others when they are feeling down, weary, and need support. The kind of compassion that gives you a break from being a superhero, no matter what the cost.

During chemotherapy, for example, we are in survival mode doing all we can to keep going. It's important to know that chemotherapy affects everyone differently, and for some, continuing regular activities and work is possible. For others, it may be nearly impossible. Whatever the situation, I encourage survivors and those around them to not judge and compare. Feeling guilty that others seem to sail through with a bubbling smile on their face isn't helpful. You are an individual with an individual physiological and psychological makeup and unique circumstances.

In our culture, we sometimes hold people up as heroes who have been diagnosed with an illness. I know I've been guilty of it. I remember people telling me I was an inspiration, and it puzzled me. All I was doing was doing the best I could to survive; I was not a hero. When that designation is given, I think we may feel obligated to live up to it and keep that brave, strong, positive face on. After all, isn't that what movies are made of?

When I look back at my experience, during treatment, I realize I did have high expectations of myself. Was it from the expectations society has about being a brave and courageous survivor? I don't know. I know I was hard on myself when I first viewed a tape of myself speaking during treatment. When I looked back and remember how much I pushed or had been hard on myself during that time, I felt compassion. I realized how hard it had been to do some of the things I had done, from speaking to working to making meals for my family, and even getting dressed for the day—nothing had been particularly easy.

Have compassion. Be there for yourself. Be there for others.

#86: Allowing others to help is a gift.

I'll never forget the first week I was diagnosed, when a fellow coach told me that when I allowed others to help, I would be giving them a gift. I struggled with this concept, as I know others do. Being independent and self-sufficient is something most of us value. However, I also know how I feel when *I* am able to help someone.

I can honestly say that experiencing the kindness of friends, family, and even strangers was one of the greatest gifts I've ever been given. And of course, expression of sincere gratitude for that support is a must!

#87: People want to help, so harness the energy by gathering a team to create the circle of support you want and need.

When going through a difficult time, the best of humanity is out in full force, reaching out to support people in need. Harnessing that energy and creating the support you want and need can be life-giving and powerful.

The ways in which this can be done are nearly limitless. Some examples are described in the sections that follow, but there is no one right way.

Special note: You may find yourself in a situation where you don't have close friends or family nearby for whatever reason. Open yourself to the possibility of kindness from those you aren't so close to. You never know when someone may have access to a wealth of support (church, organization, or otherwise) and want to reach out. And, consider special support groups at your cancer center, to connect you with others going through the same experience or with someone by phone through Imerman Angels (www.ImermanAngels.com).

For those who feel the need to be alone, keep things private, or just don't have the energy to manage it all, there are still ways to gather support that don't involve face to face interaction or a lot of time. Everyone has different needs, so it's up to you to decide what works.

Websites

In the age of electronic media, friends and loved ones across the globe can reach out and be a part of the support. Password protected websites like www.caringbridge.org or www.lotsahelpinghands.org serve many purposes.

Convenient Information Updates

Fielding phone calls and emails from friends and relatives can feel nearly impossible at a time when managing your own information, emotions, and physical well-being is challenging. Having a dedicated place where updates can be posted saves a lot of time and energy and is much better than sending mass emails and then feeling pressure to respond to them all. When not feeling up to a post, because it is online, a designated friend or family member can also post an update.

Documentation

A website can serve as a perfect way to document your journey as well as your friend's comments and words of support, all in one place, and no response is required.

Sharing Specific Needs/Wishes

Your wishes, needs, or desires can be shared to give friends, relatives, and co-workers the information and guidance as to how support you best. I've seen the posts be used to describe specific needs, such as a meal sign-up or special requests for particular types of foods/meals (appetite and nausea can play a role in what any one individual may be able to handle or desire), and/or a request for a specific prayer or thought. This type of post can be shared by a friend if you are uncomfortable doing that, and usually shares a contact number for the friend/family member who is coordinating specific support.

Email/Phone

If websites are not what you had in mind, and you are more comfortable with email, creating a group list of email contacts you want to include in your circle of support can be helpful. It may be you have the very closest of friends in one group, and then another group list where you send more general information and updates.

If technology is not for you, a designated friend can share information and updates by phone in a phone chain. Just realize that sometimes passing information one person at a time by phone can sometimes lead to misinformation being disseminated. It's similar to a game called Pass It On, in which with each passing of a secret message the information changes, and by the end it is not in any way close to the original message.

Thought and Prayer Support

The idea of asking for specific thoughts and prayers can be helpful for everyone concerned. One of the most beautiful ways of asking for specific support came from Heidi, a coaching colleague and friend, who sent this incredible email before her surgery for her mastectomy:

"Dear Friends,

As you know, my cancer surgery is scheduled for tomorrow: Friday, October 8, at noon.

In the spirit of the future I'm creating for myself, I'm writing to ask you to join my circle of support. At any time from 11:30 a.m. on, please think of me. When you do, imagine that we're together, that I'm standing next to you and we're enjoying a conversation, a joke, or a story. Wrap me in your mind in a blanket of soft yellow, the color of sunshine, my color of healing, love, and health. I will feel your energy and my body-mind will gratefully accept your gift.

With gratitude and love,

Heidi"

She shared that though these words were her own, she had learned about this through Peggy Huddleston's book, *Prepare for Surgery, Heal Faster: A Guide of Mind-Body Techniques*. Meditation techniques for relaxing to reduce anxiety before surgery, use less pain medication, and recover faster were also a part of this. She reported back to us all, less than three days after the surgery, that she had needed almost no pain medication since the morphine drip was stopped post-surgery.

The concept of creating a circle of support and asking them to think of you at a certain time, with a specific thought or prayer is powerful for both those giving and receiving.

In-Person Support

Building a list of people who want to support you by "doing something" is invaluable. People may say they want to take you to chemo, make a meal, babysit, clean your house, or just keep you company. Write down their names so you don't forget. As your treatment evolves, you may find you need more help than you thought! And don't discount people who aren't necessarily the closest of friends. New friendships can come out of this experience. And sometimes, people who aren't so close can be valuable "neutral" parties who aren't attached emotionally, and can be a nice break from family members who are and who might not be dealing well with your diagnosis.

Again, be open to the kindness of strangers. Many a meal was made for me by people from my mother's Sunday School class—people I had never met! Generosity and love is expressed in many ways, so allow it to come into your life through the kindness of strangers.

A Story of Gathering a Team

I was part of a support team, years before I was diagnosed, to a close friend with Stage IV breast cancer, who I had known since my teen years. Jean was a mother figure, about 20 years older than me, but her "support group" as she called it, was filled with younger women. She was young in spirit and loved the energy of younger women. We were her family in many ways.

It started when I moved back to North Carolina, having been gone for nearly 20 years. She had to go to radiation every day for about six weeks, and I volunteered to go with her. After doing that, she told the story of friends being jealous and wanting to share in the "fun" we had. So began her very exclusive support group. She invited special friends to be a part of this group, and we took turns taking her to chemotherapy or radiation the last five years of her life (Kristen, Ann, Anna, Gail, and me). A stuffed purple elephant, named Zoey, was also a part of the group. Zoey was able to support her when she went in to get her radiation, a place we were not allowed.

At the time, we did not know each other to speak of, though we would hear about each other through her. She started having special events or parties to bring us together every so often and thank us for supporting her, which created a bond that still exists today. The gatherings were everything from a cookout, a limo ride to a special restaurant, to a day trip to her beach house and dinner (and Zoey was always included). The gatherings were always filled with fun and laughter, bonding us in a way that helped us all when she passed away.

Who would have ever dreamed that two years after Jean's death, we would support each other, as two of us were diagnosed with breast cancer a month apart. I will always be eternally grateful to them.

#88: The most important thing to "say" is nothing. Listening is everything.

There is not one perfect thing to say to someone who is diagnosed or living with cancer, but there is one perfect thing to do: listen. It's a rare gift when another human being really listens. We all want to be heard, but there is something powerful about being allowed to express thoughts and feelings without being edited or told how to feel at a difficult time.

At the simplest level, it means resisting the urge to tell someone how to feel with clichés or other well-meaning words and instead letting them know you care and are there for them. At a more complex level, it is being fully present, giving the gift of listening with empathy that is so rare.

Listening with empathy is about being very present and in the moment, not thinking about what you are going to say next. It's about respecting the other person's experience, understanding it from their perspective without judgment, trying to fix it, or getting caught up in your own emotions. It's saying, "What you say and feel matters to me, and I hear you." It's allowing them to talk openly about their fears or challenges, without trying to stop them or make it all better. In fact, just the act of listening can make things better.

Remember, everyone wants to be heard that "This is my experience, good or bad. This is what I am feeling." Listening can acknowledge the not-so-positive emotions and give voice to them. Sometimes people stay stuck in their negative emotions because no one has bothered to listen and acknowledge their real experience. Glossing over it can make a person want to dig in more with their heels and say (mostly silently to themselves), "You don't understand, so I am going to stay here until someone finally gets what I'm experiencing!" When someone listens and understands, the lonely thoughts and feelings are given a voice that can bring relief and a path out of the darkness. Depression is not uncommon for people going through cancer treatment, and I often wonder what a difference an empathetic ear could be to them.

#89: Following a few simple tips can help you say the right thing when providing verbal support.

Sincerity, genuineness, and warmth show through, more than what you say or what your do to show support. Other than listening, a brief acknowledgement and a caring word followed by listening or an offer of support is a great place to start. Knowing they are loved and cared for by you will mean the world.

Acknowledge the situation, and let them know you are thinking of them and offer support if you are able.

If it is not a secret that they have been diagnosed or are going through treatment, acknowledge their experience. Ignoring it will make them feel like you don't care or understand. Let them know you are thinking about them, and if you want to do something for them, say so. Many people also appreciate the words, "I love you and…", "I am thinking of you," or "You will be in my thoughts/prayers," followed by a specific offer of support if you have the desire (see Sample Conversations).

Use a normal tone of voice that is sincere.

Use a voice that is empathetic and kind, but not one that sounds morbid, maudlin, or sad. Most people do not want pity. They just need to know you care.

Respond with empathy.

For example, when someone shares intimate details of the difficulties they are having or have experienced with cancer (for themselves or their family), do all in your power to keep yourself from philosophizing or offering clichés. This can unintentionally minimize their experience. Do respond with empathy, "I'm so sorry, you've been through so much. That is really hard."

Talk about everyday things.

Be sure to also talk about life in general and all you talked about before cancer—things you would normally talk about. Cancer can fill our lives, and it's good to hear normal stories.

However, don't forget to recognize and acknowledge their situation, checking in with them first. During my treatment, a friend I hadn't seen in a long time came by to see me. I was obviously hairless and very sick, but she never once asked how I was doing or acknowledged that I had cancer (like maybe, "Wow, I was so surprised to hear… how are you?"). It was strange. She talked about her life and her own challenges the entire time. My guess is that she was uncomfortable, and didn't know what to say, but ignoring the elephant in the room felt cold and distant, as she went on and on about how bad her life was.

Ask before sharing a story or information.

If you have some information you'd like to share, always ask if they want to hear about it first. "I have several resources that might be helpful, would you like to hear about them?" or "I have had experience with breast cancer, and I'm happy to share some of what I've learned if that would be helpful." However, do avoid walking up to people you barely know to share information. The number of strangers or mild acquaintances that would approach me during treatment to share information about a natural or miracle cure, offer spiritual/religious books or guidance (or question my faith/religious status), or share their bad experience with a doctor was astounding. Trust me when I say that none of this is helpful.

Share what you love and appreciate about them when appropriate.

Though you don't want it to seem like you are doing a deathbed scene and suddenly being kind, it is always uplifting to hear people share their positive experience of you. Just take the time to do what we should all do for each other. Tell them what they mean to you and how you appreciate them. Examples: "Your beauty has always shone from the inside out and always will to me." "I am so grateful for the friendship we have together." "I have always loved your honesty and your ability to make people laugh."

What to Say: Sample Conversations

Example of what you might say to someone you know socially or professionally, but may not be close to

- "Hi, Diane. I heard about your diagnosis… I'm so sorry you are having to go through this. It's a challenging time for you and your family. I just want you to know that you are in my thoughts and prayers." Then listen and let their response be your guide for what to say next. They may clearly not want to talk about it, elaborate further, or they may share that they appreciate your saying something and elaborate or stop.
- Honesty in not knowing what to say:
  - ✓ "I really don't know the right thing to say at a time like this, but I just want you to know I'm here for you…"
  - ✓ "I don't know the best thing to say at a time like this, but my heart goes out to you…I want you to know I'm keeping you close in my thoughts … ." Pause and wait for response.
- *And,* if you are in a position to help:
  - ✓ To a neighbor: "I'd really like to help out if I can. I wonder if I might be able to help by walking your dog on Saturday and Sunday or by bringing a meal over for the family this weekend?"
  - ✓ To a business associate: "I know you have that big account to service. Would it be helpful if I could help by…?"

Examples of what to say to someone with whom you are closer

Letting them know you love them and will be there through it all will feel wonderful, so try the following:

- "This just stinks." (polite version)
- "I am so sorry you are having to deal with this. This just sucks." (non-polite version, but one many can relate to, even if they are normally polite) Then, just listen and let them know you will be there for them. Listening and allowing them to vent or problem solve is invaluable.
- "I love you, and I will be here for you. We will get through this together, one day at a time..."

Examples of checking in with a friend during treatment

You: How are you? *or* How are things going today? (Said in a thoughtful, non-flippant way, but not maudlin.)

Them: I'm really tired. I just had my treatment a few days ago and am feeling a little nauseous and weak.

You: Feeling nauseous and tired is no fun. I'm sorry you are having to deal with this.

Them: It stinks. It's the hardest thing about chemo to me—having no energy. I can't do all I want to do. Things seem to be piling up.

You: It's hard to not be able to do the things you want. I'd like to help with some of those things.

Them: It is hard! There's so much we take for granted when it comes to our energy to do things. That's sweet of you to want to help.

You: What would be most helpful today, bringing your family a meal or going by the grocery store for you? *or* If I could do one thing to help you today that would have the biggest impact in making things easier, what would it be?

Them: You know, just talking to you is the best present I could possibly have today. I really appreciate you listening to me. But I do need my prescription picked up for my nausea... .

#90: Some well-meaning words of support are not helpful.

"I know how you feel…" We can never really know exactly how someone feels, even if we think we do. The implied message is that you already know how they feel, so there is no need for them to tell you how they actually feel.

"Everything is going to be all right." or *"Breast cancer is so treatable these days, and you are going to be just fine."* While these statements may be true for many women, it may or may not be true for a particular person and their situation—and there is no way of knowing the outcome. It can sound patronizing as well as minimize their situation and what they are going through.

"Aunt Agnes died of breast cancer, so you better really fight this!" Stories of pain or death are never helpful.

"Aunt Sally lived 30 years after her treatment." She may have, but she also may have had a different type of breast cancer. As shared earlier in the book, comparisons are really hard to make because there are so many different variables.

"You look great, so you must be feeling good." It's possible it may have taken hours to get ready for the day to look presentable. Energy is at an all-time low if they are going through chemotherapy. Though hair/wig and makeup may help us look good and we may be happy at the moment, there may be little correlation to our health status and how we feel inside.

"There's a reason you were diagnosed." *"This is God's will."* or *"There's a reason this happened."* Whatever your own philosophy or belief system, or theirs, it's best coming from them as to how they want to view things spiritually or philosophically. Other platitudes or clichés, are usually not helpful and are like telling someone how to think or feel. Just listen, tell them they are loved and cared about, and be there for them.

"Don't be worried about losing your hair or breast! There are more important things to focus on, like saving your life." My husband shared with a friend that I was concerned about my hair falling out. The friend said something like "She needs to be fighting for her life; that's the least of her worries! My aunt just died of breast cancer. This is serious!" Of course, it's serious, but that doesn't mean losing a body part or hair is a welcomed side effect. If you've read the book so far, this is one of many losses a survivor might experience. Let them process it in their own time.

"Think positive!"

Because this is so important to understand, both for survivors and those that care about them, I am elaborating more fully as to why this is not a helpful statement. In *It's Not About the Bike*, Lance Armstrong says, "I was coming to understand that the disease doesn't discriminate or listen to the odds; it will decimate a strong person with a wonderful attitude, while it somehow miraculously spares the weaker person who is resigned to failure. I had always assumed that if I won bike races, it made me a stronger and more worthy person. Not so."

I've met some of the most optimistic, happy, loving people I've ever known who have cancer. Though I did not know her personally, Christopher Reeve's (*Superman*) wife Dana was one of those people who exuded positivity, yet she succumbed to lung cancer in a very short time. If being positive was a cure, she would still be here.

While having hope, gratitude, and other positive emotions improve quality of life, even positive psychologists recognize the importance of negative emotions that keep us grounded, real, and honest. Researchers say the ideal balance of positive to negative emotions is a 3:1 ratio of positive to negative emotions. Emotions like sadness, anger, or grief ground us in reality and may motivate us to take action.

However, telling someone how to think or feel is where the problem lies. It might actually make them feel worse. Though most people do it as a show of support, it may send an unintended negative message that: they are not a positive person or they are not being positive (criticizing), that if they are not positive, it will impact their outcome (a myth that emotions will make tumors grow), and that it is wrong to feel the natural emotions of sadness, anger, or fear that a diagnosis can bring (making them feel bad or guilty when they do).

Having positive emotions will certainly improve quality of life, but when "being positive" means putting on a brave and happy face that is not authentic, it is not helpful.

In *The Human Side of Cancer*, one of the chapters ("The Tyranny of Positive Thinking"), Jimmie Holland discusses how urging positive thinking invalidates people's natural and understandable reactions to a threat to their lives and may keep them from getting the support they need. He also observes how many negative, pessimistic people survive their cancers and strongly urges survivors to call off the "positive attitude police."

In addition, a recent study at the Peter MacCallum Cancer Centre in Melbourne found that optimism had no impact on survival in a group of Stage IV colon cancer survivors (as it did in an earlier study with advanced lung cancer). They investigated associations between hope, optimism, anxiety, and depression in survival in patients with metastatic colorectal cancer. What they found was that quality of life, depression, and hope, all had a relationship with survival, but optimism did not (optimism as defined as a global expectation or belief that things will turn out all right). While we know that optimism can improve quality of life, in this study, it did not impact survival.

They found a very strong negative association between hope and depression, meaning essentially, the more depressed, the less hope one had. They suggest that hope might influence someone's will to seek out treatments, people, doctors, support groups, and the like that might help them live longer. Hope theory (defined by Snyder) is the belief we can impact our circumstances with a particular pathway or goal, or the will to pursue a goal with an understanding of the way to achieve it.

Because depression was a significant predictor of shortened survival, they believe that treating depression early on might impact longer survival, but more research is needed. Since more than half of breast cancer survivors experience some kind of depression, this could be important, even though the study did not include breast cancer survivors.

Bottom line: while cultivating authentic positive emotions will help improve quality of life and is very important (see Chapters 6 and 7), telling someone to be positive is not helpful and may keep them from seeking support they need, not to mention invalidating their experience and making them feel guilty and worse than they already do.

A Final Note

As the recipient of well-meaning wishes, it's important to understand that people really are doing the best they know how, and don't mean harm. Try as best you can to let comments that start to bother you roll off your back like water off a duck, be gracious, and hold on to the spirit of love that is trying to come through. As the one offering support, most people understand and appreciate that you are reaching out in the best way you know how and are grateful for your love and concern!

#91: You can show your support in a number of ways.

Stay in touch, whether by card, email, or phone.

Even when you are not confident about saying the "right" things, you can stay in touch to let them know that you are thinking of them with a heartfelt note or card, a phone call, or an email. If you only knew how much a simple "I'm thinking of you" means!

Understand that though you might not receive a thank you for the card or a reply, make no mistake: it is received and valued. Along with the feeling of being overwhelmed, fatigue, and logistics of fitting a cancer diagnosis into a person's life, responding to thoughtful notes can be nearly impossible. It's always nice to say to the recipient, "Please don't worry about responding, I know you have a lot to deal with right now."

One of the most depressing and hurtful experiences survivors share is when people they thought were good friends or even colleagues, fall off the face of the earth. While it may simply be the friend/colleague is uncertain about what to say or do, it is translated as not caring and multiplies the losses they are already feeling. So, stay in touch, even if it's just a card or email once in awhile.

Offer specific support when possible.

Be specific in offering help when possible, "Can I ___ or ____ on Tuesday?" or "I'd really like to do something that would be helpful this week, maybe pick up some groceries, make a dinner or do a load of laundry for you. Would any of those work for you?" or "I really want to help, but I'm not sure about the things that would be of most help right now." Then, list some ways you might be able to help.

Offering to babysit, cook, clean up after dinner, do other household tasks, or run an errand are all examples of helpful things to do. If they don't need help now, maybe they will next week, so keep checking in.

Don't forget that sometimes the best gift of all is that of time. Time to visit, time to laugh or cry together, to catch up, or just hang out! That, in itself, may allow you to see what support they may be needing.

Invite them to participate in all the things they did before cancer.

Everyone is different, but many people may still want to be invited to events/enjoy life. If undergoing chemotherapy, they may not want to spend time in a crowded area or feel up to it on a given day, but it's nice to know they are thought about and might welcome a dinner or a cup of coffee away from home (even in your own home).

Offer to go to their doctor or treatment visits.

It is always nice to have company when you are going to do something unpleasant. It can be a special time with a friend or loved one that can lighten the experience.

As I've tried to share throughout the book, everyone is different and has to figure out what works best for them in their situation. Some people prefer to go alone; others want a specific family member, while others want friends that lighten things up a bit for them. Some centers won't allow a friend in the infusion room, so it's important to check that out.

As a fairly independent woman, I didn't think I would need someone at first. How wrong I was. Having someone with me at chemo was important because it was usually a 12-hour day with the drive, waiting (large medical center), seeing the doctor, and then going through the infusion. I would not have been able to drive myself due to the additional drugs they sometimes gave (Benadryl®), or from the fatigue. With radiation, I easily drove myself, even though it followed months of chemotherapy. I was only in the room for a short time and needed to get back to work, so I rarely had someone go with me.

My college roommate flew from Texas to be with me on the first day of chemo. She was a take-charge, fun, proactive caregiver who was there to do all she could to make things easier for me. Her love and support meant the world to me as she supported me through my fears.

Outside of treatment, having a smart and perceptive friend or family member when going to a doctor's appointment can also be helpful as another set of ears to remember what was said, and possibly take notes for you. I took a tape recorder for some of my initial visits when my husband couldn't go so he could hear the details.

Give a practical gift that will support them.

Friends or family will sometimes offer gifts, and though they are always appreciated, they are not expected. Many new companies and websites have sprung up with perfect gifts that can be shipped immediately. The gift ideas below range from inexpensive to expensive:

- Soft mastectomy t-shirt, bra, or other surgery-related items (for time right after surgery)
- Wig headwrap, scarves, or hats
- Soft robe or nightgown
- Book or magazine
- Sleep mask
- CD of beautiful music for relaxation/meditation
- Hand sanitizer

- Gift certificate toward maid service/cleaning
- Dinner for two
- Flowers
- Digital thermometer
- DVD
- Box of special chocolates or other special treat (if you know they like this sort of thing)
- Soothing lotion
- Soft throw or small blanket to snuggle with during the day
- Exercise equipment (that they want and will use)
- Gift certificate for a wellness coach or personal trainer
- Gift certificate for an integrative medicine center's services (acupuncture, massage, and other classes)

One of the most practical and useful gifts I received that lasted into my recovery and beyond was an elliptical trainer from my mom. I had connections with used fitness equipment and was able to find a commercial grade piece that I could have in my house.

Conclusion

Support is a beautiful thing, but it is also as individual as human beings are. Survivors will find what support works best for them over time, and I encourage those around them to listen and honor whatever that may be. They may not want meals brought to the house, they may not want to be a part of a support group, they may not want to do the things *you* think are important for them. As a loved one that can be hard. But what I know for sure is that as a survivor/patient, the most important and wonderful gift of all will be just knowing that people will be there for you, with love through it all.

Chapter References

Fredrickson, B. (2009). *Positivity*. New York: Crown Publishers.

Holland, J.C. & Lewis, S. (2000). *The Human Side of Cancer: Living With Hope, Coping With Uncertainty*. New York: HarperCollins.

Imerman Angels
www.ImermanAngels.org.

Snyder, C.R. (1989). Hope theory: Rainbows of the mind. *Psychological Inquiry*. 13: 249–275.

9

Survivorship

Hope is like the sun, which, as we journey towards it,
casts the shadow of our burden behind us.
—Samuel Smiles

Remember that it is our choice, and ours alone,
to turn even a nightmare into a positive experience.
—Elizabeth Kubler-Ross

Survivor. Cancer survivor. How did that happen to me? And I'm guessing if you are reading this, you are wondering how it happened to you, too. Yet, I am the face of cancer. You or your loved one is the face of cancer. One of every three women and one of every two men will have had cancer in their lifetime. It is something we should not be ashamed of as in years gone by, but grateful for. Treatments have brought us this far, and we are surviving a cancer diagnosis.

That is why the word "survivor" has come to be. Our country has nearly 12 million cancer survivors of all types because we now have various treatment options that allow us to live longer and manage this disease. Regardless of the cancer of origin, we are all cancer survivors in a community that has lived to tell their story. I have been fortunate to meet some of the most amazing, inspirational people I've ever known through this community, and I am grateful for each one.

In the beginning, I was not comfortable with the term "survivor," especially during treatment, as I felt I was very much a patient and had not survived the experience. And I didn't fully appreciate what the word meant. A part of me didn't like the less-than-positive label that implied, barely hanging on or surviving and not thriving. As such, many survivors have embraced the word "thriver" in its place. For me, "thriver" describes the renewed zest and appreciation for life after treatment, but it may not fully capture the entire experience. "Thrivership" is a double-edged sword given the continuing side effects one may live with. On the upside, we are often doing much more than surviving as we have chosen to take our circumstances and "thrive" despite the challenges. Yet on the downside, the impact of cancer treatment can sometimes reverberate for years, as no part of our lives is left untouched.

Though I do not like labels, I have now come to understand the need to describe this evolving state of the cancer experience. "Survivor" seems to be the most accepted term for the moment, and most importantly, identifies an amazing group of people I have come to know and love, and I accept it.

Living as a survivor can mean many things, from learning to live with a new reality, dealing with fears and anxiety around the possibility of recurrence, uncertainty, late or long-term side effects from treatment, long-term medications with their own side effects, ongoing medical appointments, and can even mean living *with* cancer and its treatment for the remainder of their lives.

In this chapter, I share some information and issues around survivorship that may explain the unique place in which we find ourselves. Much beauty is found in the world of survivors, and their experiences can be inspiring. I end the book with the grief, grace, gratitude, and hope that encompass our world.

#92: Survivorship is a term used to describe the growing world of cancer survivors.

Many years ago, cancer was a death sentence, but as treatments have become more effective, nearly 12 million survivors (of all types) are living in the United States. However, as noted in previous sections, treatment that has saved a life may also impact quality of life and future health. The National Cancer Institute (NCI) under the National Institutes of Health (NIH) created a branch dedicated to cancer survivorship. The Office of Cancer Survivorship was established in 1996 by the National Cancer Institute to support and promote research that examines and addresses the long- and short-term effects of cancer and its treatment. The awareness of the needs of survivors were highlighted even more in a 2006 book from the Institute of Medicine and National Research Council of the National Academies entitled, *From Cancer Patient to Cancer Survivor: Lost in Transition*, a large book which detailed the numerous short-term and late effects from cancer and its treatment.

Understanding this world of survivorship has become a booming area of research and program development to address the needs of survivors in order to impact their quality of life. In fact, there is a movement to form a new branch of oncology called survivorship medicine.

#93: You are a survivor from the time of diagnosis throughout the remainder of life.

The National Coalition for Cancer Survivorship (NCCS) pioneered the definition "survivorship," which has been commonly agreed upon and utilized by most organizations. Years ago, the word "victim" was often used to describe someone diagnosed. Thank goodness that has changed. The NCCS has expanded the definition to include family, friends, and caregivers affected by the diagnosis as well.

Macmillan Cancer Support in the United Kingdom defines a cancer survivor as someone who is "living with or beyond cancer" and has completed the initial cancer treatment, is living with the disease but not in the terminal phases, or has had cancer in the past.

Among survivors, the term brings up varied emotional responses and opinions, though it is embraced widely as a positive, descriptive term. Still, a more positive term is embraced by many, calling themselves "thrivers." They say they are not just surviving and holding on, but *thriving*. Still, some don't feel they are survivors until after initial treatment ends, some want the experience to be behind them, while others say they don't want to be defined and labeled by cancer.

Voices of Survivors, a non-profit and website of the same name (www.voicesofsurvivors.org), celebrates these voices in an extremely positive light, with individuals describing what it means to be a survivor in their own terms and using their own definition(s).

Over the years, I have heard a variety of interesting responses regarding the label. Some of the varied responses include an 11-year breast cancer survivor who remarked, "I don't consider myself a survivor, just lucky." While another says, "I always cringe when people tell me I am cured or that I am a survivor. I know those undetectable cells are lurking in my body... Treatment bought me a few years, though the first five were not pleasant due to side effects from medication. Most doctors I see remain super vigilant, and I am constantly being confronted with scary moments..." Another individual rejected the term survivor, as implying heroism or bravery, saying the merit badge for just living through the treatment of a disease was not deserved. On the other hand, an embracing comment from one woman was that the term "survivor" was empowering to people fighting the disease, believing that it represented a positive mindset.

Whether one chooses to embrace the word survivor or would just as soon put it all behind them is an individual decision, with no right or wrong answer. I agree that the term "survivor" is not perfect, yet having a term is important to describe the altered health status we encounter after treatment. It's also important to note that people used to be ashamed and not let those around them know they had cancer (and some still don't, especially in other parts of the world), so being a proud survivor is also saying, "I'm not ashamed of what happened to me, and I am the face of cancer," to help reduce the stigma and create awareness.

On the other hand, this term often brings people together in a positive way. Being able to support each other and advocate for our needs as a large community, can make all of our lives better. I advocate for all survivors, regardless of the type of cancer or chronic disease they may have, as we have many experiences that are similar.

#94: A survivorship care plan is important to have when you finish treatment.

It is important to have a survivorship care plan that you put together with your health care team. A survivorship care plan is a comprehensive summary and plan that communicates the details of treatment you have had, with recommendations for follow-up care and monitoring after formal treatment ends. The Institute of Medicine (IOM) report (see #92) made a series of recommendations of what should be included in that plan.

It should include a complete record of treatments so you can share with your primary care providers as you transition away from treatment. It should summarize potential late effects, their symptoms and treatment, recommendations for screening, psychosocial effects, and how to manage them and/or identify symptoms of other serious health issues that may arise as a result of treatment. Many organizations are beginning to have their own versions, but many do not. For example, if you visit www.livestrongcareplan.org, you can develop an individualized care plan that you can review and discuss with your health care team. You may need information from them in order to fully complete the plan, so check the website to see what you will need.

Guidelines from the IOM include recommendations for a healthy lifestyle or wellness plan in the survivorship plan. It is important for doctors to communicate what is important in terms of lifestyle to reduce risk for other diseases and/or recurrence as a first step.

Recommendations for healthy living are important. However, I know that information or a plan someone else designs doesn't necessarily change behavior. It's like writing a New Year's resolution for someone, without their input and with no specific plan to achieve it. As I've shared before, I encourage you to meet with a health or wellness coach to put together a plan with these recommendations that is alive and flexible, yet realistic and sustainable, that will help you work toward optimal well-being, one step at a time.

#95: Survivors live with varying amounts of fear and anxiety about recurrence.

Managing fear of cancer recurrence is one of the top three needs survivors have, according to the Breast Cancer Registry. Living with the risk of recurrence changes the way most of us think and live. The task of learning to live with the unknown can be a difficult one at first, dealing with the uncertainty and managing fear and anxiety that comes.

At the end of cancer treatment, anxiety is often high because "doing" something for management of the cancer, such as consistency of treatment (chemotherapy, radiation, etc.), is over. Many may feel that our bodies betrayed us once and the potential persists for this to happen again.

I was at a social event recently, and met a breast cancer survivor who was years out from her treatment of a lumpectomy and radiation. My husband shared that I was writing a book and that I was a breast cancer survivor. Her eyes welled up with tears as she shared that she didn't talk about her breast cancer because she felt like if she talked about it, it would come back. And I'll never forget meeting a woman the year of my treatment at a Sister's Network meeting who shared that she had not spoken of her breast cancer for seven years, until that very day, let alone spoken of her fear of recurrence.

Sometimes, people talk about it openly, while others keep it hidden away and never share. Whether survivors talk about it or not, it is a reality that doesn't go away. The first step to dealing with the fear and anxiety is to identify it, name it, and call it what it is. I had never known the kind of feeling I felt when treatment ended. It showed up as a gnawing in my stomach that would not go away. I did not know what it was about. I was excited that treatment was over and was ready to get my life going again, yet I had this anxious feeling in my body I'd never experienced before. I don't mean I'd never been afraid or unsure in my life—this was different. When a counselor at the cancer center said that I was learning how to deal with "a new reality" (or "new normal" that is often used), it annoyed me. What did that mean exactly? I wanted my old reality back. I now understand that the world as I had known it had a lot of certainty, and cancer changed that. My body knew it before my mind did. It was an enormous shift for my mind and body to have to deal with.

As the years have passed, anxiety has lessened. I find there is less talk about it among my survivor friends, though it is always in the back of our minds. An ache is never just a getting-older-ache or pain. Each new physical issue requires a careful and patient evaluation. Even regular check-ups bring anxiety.

We sometimes call the feeling around routine or diagnostic (a problem has arisen) imaging "scanxiety." As survivors, we learn that interruptions come. Sometimes, our days and lives aren't always as we've planned them to be because of a new concern. Taking time to deal with what is most important in the moment and finding the goodness, beauty, and light in the day in spite of it becomes our task. Dealing with the interruption that a concern represents is one thing, but waiting for the test results is quite another. Quelling anxiety can become our most challenging task.

Overall, being able to manage worry and anxiety about recurrence is important to live life fully and in the present, "keeping the elephant small." Cancer is the "elephant" in the room that represents the possibility of cancer returning, always in the back of our minds. For everyone, that fear and anxiety will be in varying amounts, but it is there whether it is large or very small. The good news is that it does gradually get smaller as each month and year passes.

What You Can Do

- Be in control of what you can in regards to your health: make healthy lifestyle habits a part of your daily routine (stop smoking, lose weight, etc.), take medications that reduce your risk, focus on the life you have and the things that bring you peace and happiness
- Enjoy and be in the present. When we find ourselves worrying, chances are we are in the past or the future, instead of appreciating the now. Think about things you are grateful for when you are feeling fearful or anxious, which can shift your thinking.
- Practice building positive emotions as discussed in Chapters 6 and 7.
- Find things to do that give you a sense of purpose and meaning, like helping others.
- Meditate or pray, connecting to your spirituality or higher power (God).
- Express your fears with a trusted, empathetic friend or counselor.
- Understand that some things are out of our control, and find peace in doing what you can—and surrender the rest.

I have also watched friends live life fully *with* cancer, or recurrence, for many years. I have found that an acceptance of my mortality and knowing that, if it did return, I would be okay. As Elizabeth Edwards spoke so eloquently about her recurrence, she used the phrase, "Though my days might be shorter than they otherwise would have been..." It resonated with me. None of us are guaranteed another day. We hope we will have more than less, but all we can do is live life fully each day, with all the presence and savoring we can.

#96: Survivors live with a sense of uncertainty and a heightened sense of mortality.

As a result of this fear of recurrence, most of us live with a sense of uncertainty. Typically, no one thinks that cancer was going to happen in the first place, but when it does, it shifts a paradigm from being certain about how life will progress, to the reality that we don't know and that life is uncertain. It is an unsettling feeling at first, taking away the security we often grow up with, that things in life are certain.

The understanding that life is fragile becomes clear. Uncertainty about being guaranteed another day, year, or decade shrouds our path, because we have learned we can't be certain of many things. As time passes from treatment, the intensity may change, but it impacts the way we live our lives going forward.

The first year after treatment ended, I remember signing a one-year contract for a health club membership and how uncertain it felt. Would I be here in a year? It may sound silly, but that is an example of how real it was at the time.

The truth is that none of us know when our lives will end. However, for cancer survivors, there is renewed and heightened awareness around our mortality. When a life-threatening disease lurks in the shadows with the chance of a return, and with no particular rhyme or reason, people can't help but live with a heightened awareness of their mortality.

This may, in turn, lead to new directions in a survivor's life. Many people will say they don't have time for small or petty things anymore. They don't want to spend time around people or places that don't support them or a meaningful, positive existence. "Living large" or "living out loud" can become the motto because we have learned none of us are promised another day.

#97: The downside of cancer is not a pretty pink ribbon.

Similar to a title to a keynote I did early in my survivorship, "Grief, Grace, and Gratitude," I wanted to try to capture or summarize the journey of being a survivor from this point to the end the book with the aspects of grief, grace, gifts, gratitude, and hope we feel as survivors.

As from Gilda's quote in Chapter 6, though there are gifts, there is a downside. Sometimes, the public is focused on the pretty pink ribbon without fully understanding the downside it represents. Despite the many women who will now live because of emerging treatments, many will die, and others will live with long-term health issues. I lost a treasured friend, years before my own diagnosis. Yes, breast cancer still takes beautiful, loving women in the prime of their lives. That is difficult.

It is a mixed bag, for sure, as I've shared throughout these pages. Some people will say it's the best thing that ever happened to them, while others are angry for the devastation it may have caused in their life (divorce, significant physical long-term side effects, etc.). I fall somewhere closer to the positive side, but it is no doubt mixed.

While I would never want to go back to who I was before cancer, I think I could have done without it, thank you, though I appreciate what cancer has taught me. The gifts are enormous. As with all pain and challenges in life, we grow when we embrace and learn from them. We can come out on the other side better, stronger, wiser, and richer for the experience. Through brokenness and sorrow, we grow and become more resilient, flourishing with renewed purpose and meaning.

My own health changed forever when I was diagnosed with breast cancer. Because I had always been so healthy, and had worked so hard to keep it that way, watching my body age and weaken was hard. Many look at me and say, "But you are so healthy, what do you mean?" I have fought hard to deal with the altered health status I've found myself in over the last seven years, though I am grateful to be here and as healthy as I am. Between surgeries, medicine, hormone-blocking treatments, hysterectomy, chronic UTIs leading to intestinal infection (clostridium difficile), to osteopenia, and other setbacks too numerous to mention, it has been a journey of recovery with each successive issue.

For me, it has also represented embracing a continuous, purposeful fight to regain my health and reduce risk of recurrence or other disease, with resilience and resolve toward this daily mission.

#98: Amazing grace gives us life.

In one definition of grace from Webster's, "The exercise of love, kindness, mercy, favor; disposition to benefit or serve another; favor bestowed or privilege conferred," captures the spirit and gifts that my experience as a survivor has given me. The generosity and kindness of spirit, the blessings, the support in weathering the storm, and the love from humanity (and God) I have felt on this journey have been undeserving. I will be forever grateful for the grace bestowed upon me. I will continue to share that which was so freely given to me and pay it forward.

#99: The gifts of joy, meaning, and purpose fill our lives.

A renewed sense of joy in celebrating what matters in life and the consciousness of savoring each moment, the small things in life, are some of the greatest gifts that come from being a survivor. Some of the most meaningful and joyful moments of my life have been because of the connections and moments made with other cancer survivors, many of whom have devoted their lives to making life better for others who have been diagnosed with cancer. Their lives are full with passion and purpose. Survivorship often gives a renewed sense of meaning and purpose in giving back.

My own diagnosis immediately sparked a passion to share what I had learned about early detection so I could save others from the same path. In my mail program, I named a file "Pam's Passion," describing the work I began soon after being diagnosed. It began with an article I wrote about my experience for a local magazine entitled "Cancer Will Never Happen to Me." The response to that article let me know there was a need and I had to keep talking. I continued to speak during my treatment about early detection and later created a website to share the information. (www.knowyourdensity. com).

It has also meant giving back to those who had been through challenging times with their health and well-being because I knew all too well what it was like, and because of that understanding, I could not turn my back and forget. Creating the first program of wellness coaching for cancer survivors meant that many people would not know of its value, so three years of my life was dedicated as a coach and co-investigator in research (a labor of love) to show its efficacy.

It's meant giving back by advocating for survivors in becoming a LIVE**STRONG** leader and delegate, participating in events at the state, national, and international level for this and other organizations. It's meant volunteering on boards, committees and focus groups, speaking, advocating, and planning for positive changes for survivors and patients of all kinds. Many survivors, like me, fill our lives with this type of meaning and purpose by giving back in these ways.

We often have an urgency to advocate and/or make life better for others after a diagnosis. I am one of thousands. But others sometimes say, "Get over the cancer thing…move on!" And I say, that's fine; to each his own. However, if it weren't for survivors becoming impassioned to make a difference, nothing would ever change. Thank goodness for people like Lance Armstrong who didn't turn his back after surviving. Thank goodness for all of the survivors who devote their time and talents in volunteering or starting organizations or companies that advocate and support us all!

#100: Being a survivor engenders gratitude.

Survivorship means gratitude for so many things. It's gratitude for the people who dedicate their careers to the cancer world, from the researcher, doctor, nurse, advocate, and navigator, to the volunteer. It's gratitude for all those who helped us and are helping us through this journey. It's gratitude for the gift of another day to do all the things that make up a life.

Personally, it's gratitude for being able to see my sons graduate from high school and college and supporting them as they move into adulthood. It's the gift of watching my son get married and experiencing the love and friendship of a daughter-in-law. It's the renewed closeness to my husband of over 30 years. It's the friendships of other survivors, whose loving spirits I am privileged to know and friends and family who have helped me along the journey.

#101: Hope is more than a wish and plays an important role in our survivorship.

As survivors, hope is what we have to cling to—that we will have another day, another year, another decade, or half century. Hope is more than a wish; it's a life filled with plans and dreams that keep us going to the next mountaintop. It's doing all we can to take care of ourselves so we will be here to experience the large and small things that make up a life.

I have had the privilege of knowing some incredibly inspiring survivors, who by their journey and view of the world have inspired hope in me. That hope is about how they live life joyfully and fully, in spite of either a diagnosis that seemed so dire or a prognosis that would have left most with no place for hope. I have been very close to several Stage IV cancer survivors, and all of them were/are an inspiration to me.

One of them, Suzanne Lindley, was diagnosed with Stage IV colon cancer at the young age of 32. Watching her live her life without boundaries, despite seemingly insurmountable odds with cancer "here, there, and everywhere" (as she puts it), has given me hope in this journey.

The following update was shared on her wedding anniversary last year that captures the hopefulness and journey of survivors everywhere:

"Today, Ronnie and I celebrate 24 years of marriage. Our vows have been put to the test in these two dozen years...for better or worse (most better), for richer and poorer (a bit of both), and in sickness and health (just imagine). We have spent exactly half of these years without cancer. The other half in its wake.

We have waded through the thick and thin of life, shared tender moments, heartbreaking losses, inspiring friendships, courageous encounters, and more wonderful memories than many people ever dream to see.

We've watched our families endure, our daughters grow, and our friends rally. The important things...they are the simplest and fade all too quickly. The first wobbly steps of a toddler turn quickly into the confident steps of a young adult. We have been lucky. This disease taught us about fragility, but forced us to find strength. While other families wanted life moments to speed up, we tried to slow ours down. We've cherished and appreciated the change of seasons.

Hopes and plans...not always as we expect them to be. Twelve years ago, we traded thoughts of expanding our family to stretching time. Days have turned into weeks, weeks to months, and months to years...as we started looking forward to college graduations, someday weddings, and future grandchildren—an adorable toddler found her way into our lives. Today, of all days, a dream put to rest has been fulfilled. Fate stepped in and we are not only celebrating the anniversary of our wedding but the addition of Chloe.

She is two years old, 36 inches tall, 34 pounds, brown curly hair, big brown eyes, and talkin' up a storm!! So...it's officially Chloe day!"

Suzanne started a non-profit to help anyone diagnosed with tumors that have spread to the liver, called "YES! Beat Liver Tumors." I am in awe of the work she has done and the hope she has inspired around the world. She personifies the word, both in her work and her personal life.

Before my own diagnosis, my friend Jean Pendergraft lived with Stage IV breast cancer for nearly 16 years. As the free spirit and artist she had become as a result of her diagnosis, she showed me how someone could make her life special in the smallest of moments and dance in the rain, in spite of incredible challenge. She loved her life and everything in it. She would often say, "Nobody needs to feel sorry for me. I have a wonderful life!"

So hope is more than just a wish for survivors. Hope is a passion for living and anticipation of the next beautiful milestone, planning for it, and appreciating each step. May we all learn to find the beauty in each moment, and should it rain, may we remember to dance!

Life is not about waiting for the storms to pass.
It's about learning how to dance in the rain!
—Anonymous

Chapter References

Beat Liver Tumors
  www.BeatLiverTumors.org

The Cancer Support Community
  www.csc.BreastCancerRegistry.org

Hewitt, M., Greenfield, S., & Stovall, E. [Eds.]. (2006). *From Cancer Patient to Cancer Survivor: Lost in Transition.* Washington, D.C.: National Academies Press.

Society for Women's Health Research. (2005). Life After Early Breast Cancer: Science, Perceptions & Communication Surrounding Risk of Recurrence.

Epilogue

It came in the final weeks of preparing to submit my final manuscript of this book to the publisher: I found a mass under my arm. I couldn't believe it. This was not happening. The chaos I felt in my "knowing" mind and body was overwhelming.

It was Friday morning, July 8, 2011, the day I had planned to finally submit this book I'd been working on for two years, when I received a phone call confirming my intuition. This call was just the "abnormal results" call, but I had known from the moment I felt it, that it was cancer. The call was just more confirmation.

The wait had been agonizing. The anxiety, trying to put it in the back of my mind while continuing to live, adding to the list of an already busy life with my dad's cancer diagnosis, my mom having two unexpected surgeries, my work, scheduling tests, and waiting yet again for results. Just wanting to know so I could *do* something about it was the hardest part of all. But I had to wait some more.

This is the life I speak of in this book. We live our lives with uncertainty from day to day, knowing that cancer could return and that with each new test and result we receive, our lives are hanging in the balance. Waiting in the space of *I know, but I hope I don't know, but what if it is*, reality can be daunting. This life changes you for better or for worse. It's the reason we learn to live our lives out loud. None of us are promised another day. We just happen to have the gift of knowing that.

On the following Monday, July 11, minutes before my biopsy, I ironically submitted my book through the Duke server (via the Internet), the place where I spent nearly a year in treatment seven years earlier.

About two days later, my suspicions were undeniably confirmed when I heard the dreaded words again: "I'm sorry. It's cancer."

As we bring the final details of this book to a close, I am in a hopeful place. We are hopefully shrinking a tumor with oral medication, but I won't know until the results of the next scan.

Rather than rewrite/add to sections of the book and delay its release, I have decided to end it here and through my speaking and future writing, I will share more of my story. I am certain to write about it in my blog. So if you would like to follow the rest of the story, please go to www.PamSchmid.com.

Blessings, peace, and love to all.

Appendix:
Cancer Will Never Happen to Me

The emotional and physical journey of a healthy person diagnosed with breast cancer.

**Written by Pam Whitt Schmid
for the September/October 2004 issue of *Cary Magazine*.**

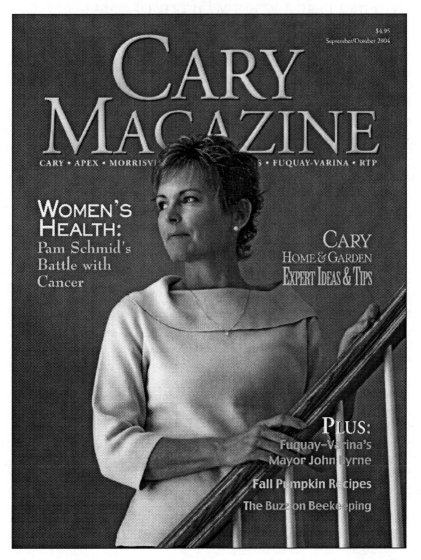

Reprinted with permission: *Cary Magazine*, Western Wake County, North Carolina

Cancer Will Never Happen to Me

The emotional and physical journey of a healthy person diagnosed with breast cancer.

Written By Pam Whitt Schmid, Wellness Coach and Personal Trainer

Let's see. Here's the list:

Non-smoker

Exercise five days a week

Eat a low-fat, balanced diet

Low total cholesterol level in the 140s

Avoid hormones

Breast fed both children

No caffeine

No family history

"Real age" of 34 based on health exam

OK. That should do it. No cancer for me ... or so I thought. I'm 46 years old, a health and fitness professional of 23 years and am being treated aggressively for an invasive, Stage II breast cancer. I never looked sick before my diagnosis and had the energy of a 20 year old, yet I had multiple cancerous tumors growing inside of me, threatening my life. And now, all the health I have enjoyed for years has given way to a flip side of my worst fears and nightmares. I have no reason to have breast cancer. People tell me how vulnerable it makes them feel. I understand. If I can get cancer, anyone can.

As you can imagine, I have learned more than I ever wanted to know since my diagnosis. I thought I knew what there was to know after losing a close friend to breast cancer a few years ago. I hope that in sharing what I've learned, as well as my emotional roller coaster, myths will be dispelled about breast cancer, its treatment and effects as a patient and why we all need to push for answers. The overriding truth is that there is still so much we don't know. Survival rates are improving, but women are still dying needlessly in the prime of their lives.

Before I begin, I want to share an analogy for what my diagnosis and prognosis felt like: We're going to line up 10 of you to jump off this very rocky cliff. We know it's scary, and you are scared of heights, but you have to do this in order to live. At least two of you are going to die, but not immediately. You'll all suffer quite a bit before that happens, but you won't know if you are one of the ones that are going to die. We don't know how long your life will be interrupted, but your mind and body will never be the same. Now, it's important to think positive. Don't get discouraged because the odds are in your favor. Get ready, JUMP!

The only way to describe my emotional reaction is to say that it went from one extreme to the other on a day-to-day basis. Days seemed liked years initially. Mastectomy? Chemo? Radiation? I could die? Me? No way. I can't have cancer. This is just a bad dream. Why now, when my professional life has never been more exciting and all my hard work is starting to pay off? Most importantly, I don't have time for this! My growing business had just been spotlighted on WTVD and WRAL. I'd just been asked to serve as co-chair for a newly formed American College of Sports Medicine committee on health, fitness and wellness coaching.

Discovering the Cancer

It was April 12, the day before a special trip with Wellcoaches to the American College of Sports Medicine conference in Orlando, when I received the call. It was 8 a.m. on a Monday morning when the doctor called to say, "The radiologist called in this report a few minutes ago because they think you have breast cancer. You need to see a breast surgeon right away. Do you have the name of a surgeon I can call to get you in with?" Sure, right in my back pocket.

My close friend who passed away a few years ago had a support group of friends of which I was a part. We had now become friends. Ironically, one of those women had been diagnosed with an early stage cancer a month earlier, so I quickly called her for a number, thinking how bizarre that three out of the six of us had breast cancer.

My husband happened to be home that morning and watched on in horror as I quickly dialed multiple numbers and went from call to call. When I finally got off the phone, we both looked at each other in shock and then embraced each other, crying.

Within two hours I was in a surgeon's office. The report was clear. All the signs pointed to cancer. There were small groups of calcifications that didn't look right, plus the size and shape of the tumor (only one at this point, but stay tuned) looked like cancer. I had no idea they could tell with such certainty, just by a report. We scheduled a mammotome biopsy for the next week.

Six months earlier, in October, I had found something in my right breast that turned out to be a simple fluid-filled cyst. I was a bit surprised when the doctor called me the week after and said they were concerned about some calcifications in my left breast and wanted me to follow up in six months. I was in my car, and remember thinking how odd it was that the doctor was spending a lot of time telling me about this, and how I shouldn't worry about it. I had NO idea. I wasn't worried, since the other lump was fluid filled and no problem, this probably wasn't either.

But, I went home, and started feeling around. I found a pebble-like mass that did not feel right. It felt like what I'd heard people describe as cancer. I went in to the doctor several weeks later for him to check it out. He said I could go to a breast surgeon if I wanted, but he didn't think it was anything, and we could check it at the follow up visit in April.

Well, ignorance is bliss, if only for a short time. Why would I want to pursue it further if he didn't think it was a problem and the ultrasound on the other lump was negative? I had no reason to have breast cancer. I thought I would be overreacting to go to a surgeon, for heaven's sake. Now, I know that the best thing I could have done would have been to see a breast surgeon. They see cancer every day and know much more about breast lumps than a gynecologist. Hindsight is always 20/20.

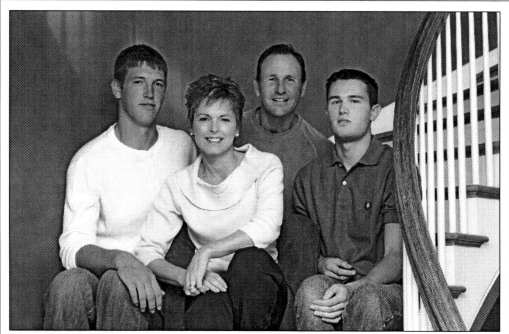

The Schmid family and Pam's support system (l to r): Jeremy, Pam, Jerry and Dustin.

The scariest part of all is that I may never have known I had cancer had I not been persistent on that fateful day in April. It was my follow-up visit six months later, where my doctor had ordered a diagnostic mammogram. I was in the dressing room waiting for the radiologist to look at the mammogram film when the technician came in and said, "You can go home now." I said, "What about the ultrasound? I'm supposed to get an ultrasound, plus I'm being billed for it." She said, "Oh, we've taken it off the bill already." I said, "Well, what about this lump?" "You have a lump? I didn't know you had one, where is it? Let me feel it. Oh. OK. I'll be right back."

She then led me back to the ultrasound room. What if I'd just said, "OK" and left? I didn't think I had cancer. I wasn't really concerned. It would have been really easy to leave. Remember, the mammogram never showed the tumors; the ultrasound did.

> "*I* have no reason to have breast cancer If I can get cancer anyone can."

Usually, a woman has to find a lump, tell her doctor and THEN a "diagnostic mammogram" is ordered (translation: ultrasound or other appropriate imaging). Three years before I found the lump, I remember arguing with the technician that I wanted an ultrasound. She tried to explain that my doctor had not ordered it, and that I didn't have a lump, so they couldn't do it. I'd been told in my 30s I had "dense breasts," and my experiences before had always included an ultrasound. I knew I needed one, but didn't totally understand why. So I left that day and didn't get another mammogram until three years later. I wonder what they would have found that day had they done ultrasounds on both breasts. They say cancer grows for years before we can feel them.

If you have ever been told after a mammogram that you have dense breast tissue, as a majority of pre-menopausal women and women from all age groups have, you must be diligent with self exam and follow up any palpable lump and insist on an ultrasound or other diagnostic screening, because tumors are difficult, if not impossible, to see on a mammogram. Routine use (without a palpable lump) of ultrasound is being studied, but its use varies from state to state and between facilities. So why do we bother going through the torture of a mammogram if you

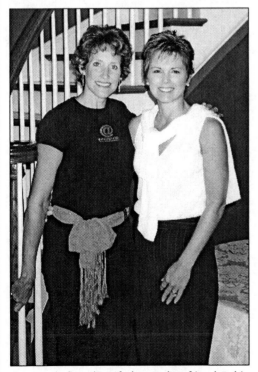

On Pam's first day of chemo, her friend Robin Burch, a former roommate while at the University of Texas at Austin, came to be with her for support.

"*The* scariest part of all is that I may never have know I had cancer had I not been persistent on that fateful day in April. "

have dense breasts? They do show telltale signs of cancer in the form of small, unusual groups of calcifications. Even ultrasounds aren't perfect.

After going to Duke Hospital for a second opinion, they did an MRI of both breasts. They picked up multiple tumors. Yes, tumors with an s. I had tumors in multiple quadrants of my breast. The MRI also did not accurately reflect the final pathology, but it showed more than the ultrasound. My final pathology from the mastectomy, showed tumors with sizes of 4.5 centimeters, 1.3, 1.2, and 0.8 centimeters, all much larger than any test had shown. Any one of them would have been significant. Remember knowledge is power and life saving. Don't rely solely on technology to find a problem. Trust your intuition and be diligent. Don't wait. Early detection can save your life.

Because of my age and the nature of my cancer, an aggressive approach was necessary. Without treatment I'd have a little more than 50 percent chance of living 10 years; with treatment about 80 percent. The treatment plan included the mastectomy, four months of chemotherapy with Adriamycin/Cytoxan/Taxol every two weeks followed by radiation for about six weeks, another surgery to complete my reconstruction, then hormonal therapy for the next 10 years. My surgeon told me she would need to watch me very closely over the next five years.

Learning How to be a Cancer Patient

So how does someone who has always put health as a priority and spent most of her life trying to prevent major disease take all this? It's like investing your life savings in stock market and losing it all at once.

Knowing how to be sick is not one of my better qualities. My first day of chemotherapy was especially traumatic only because I was surrounded by very sick people and I wondered how long it would take before I looked like them. A few doctors told me that they think it's particularly hard on people who are healthy and well because they aren't used to being sick. I don't like taking medicines, needles or having surgery, and I don't do well with anesthesia.

Since April, I have had two mammotone biopsies (in-office procedures), one sentinel node biopsy (requires going under), which required drains being put in after two weeks from the seroma pain, MRIs, CT body scans, genetic testing, blood work, mastectomy with reconstruction and drains for three long weeks (felt like having a stick under my skin that wrapped from under my arm and around my chest), recovery from major surgery, chemotherapy every two weeks and give myself daily shots.

I have a team of doctors now. I have a medicine cabinet full of medicines and products to deal with side effects from chemotherapy. How's that for a health and wellness experience! It's not what I had in mind, but you learn to deal with what has been handed to you. What other choice is there?

People often tell cancer patients to stay positive or that attitude is everything. I've always been an optimist, eternally hopeful in the dimmest of situations. I have experienced a lot in my life, both good and bad, and I've never said "why me?" Life happens. I am dealing with what is being thrown my way the best I can. I have good days. I have bad days. I'm an optimistic person by nature and will continue to be so. But isn't it OK for me to be sad once in a while? And isn't it possible that it's healthy to go through a grieving process? I'm optimistic but I'm not a saint!

The most helpful comments to me have been from a friend who has dealt with chronic disease for years, and her words of empathy are validating. "I know it's hard, this is really the pits," or empathizing comments in nature. It's not pity; its understanding and

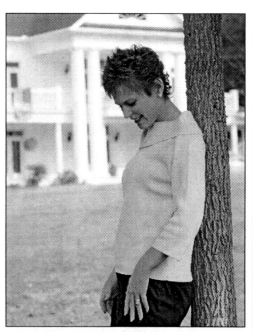

Pam lives in Clayton in what she describes as "a Southern belle's dream." She is a self-described Scarlett O'Hara, mostly because she took the curtains to make a ball gown, taking a small budget to design and build the house herself. Pam said the project was one of the biggest challenges of her life until her battle with cancer.

acknowledging that what you are dealing with is challenging! To do otherwise is to minimize its significance.

I have also discovered that most people don't know a lot about breast cancer and its treatment. I was in that category myself. The generalities and comparisons are sometimes frustrating as a patient because there are too many details and variables to compare. Below are some facts that might be helpful to understand about cancer and the patient:

- All breast cancers are not the same. There are five main stages. The first stage, 0, is not life threatening. Usually treatment involves a lumpectomy and possible radiation. It raises your risk of an invasive cancer, a potentially life threatening cancer. Stages 1-4 are invasive and have the potential to spread to organs. There are different types of invasive cancers that respond to different treatments. The stages and the type determine the aggressiveness of treatment.

- Cancer can spread even though it's not in the lymph nodes. Between 20-30 percent of the time it spreads through the bloodstream.

- There is never a 100-percent cure or assurance that the cancer has not spread. Even after aggressive treatment, there is no test to find micro-metastatic spread in the body. Current tests show "gross" cancers that have grown large enough to see. Cancer can lie dormant and come back many years down the road.

- The side effects of chemo are much more than just fatigue and nausea. The details are of such a tedious nature that they are saved for the poor, unfortunate close friends or family who have to hear about them. Chemotherapy kills

"Remember, knowledge is power and life saving. Don't rely solely on technology to find a problem. Trust your intuition and be diligent. Don't wait. Early detection can save your life."

all rapidly dividing cells, both good and bad, which affects all major systems of the body. Problems range from anemia, central nervous system problems, infection, blood clotting problems, mouth and throat problems, digestive system problems and bone and joint pain.

- Women who have had mastectomies and/or lymph nodes removed are at increased risk for a problem called lymphedema. It can cause permanent swelling of the arm. Special garments/ sleeves must be worn during air travel, exercise or other changes in pressure. Lymphedema can occur suddenly, even up to 20 years post surgery.

- With some treatments, you lose the hair on your head (Adriamycin) and all other hair, including eyebrows and eyelashes (Taxol).

- If the patient is pre-menopausal and going through chemotherapy, most go through immediate menopause, which is severe in nature. What occurs naturally over a decade or so, happens within months. Hot flashes, insomnia, night sweats, skin changes, etc.

- Muscle loss in the large muscle groups (legs/hips) occurs unless strength training is done regularly throughout treatment.

- Adriamycin will cause permanent heart damage, but may not show up clinically, meaning it may or may not cause a problem. Taxol often causes permanent neuropathy, numbness and tingling in the hands or feet.
- Bone loss occurs causing a higher risk for osteoporosis.
- Short-term memory loss happens so often; we call it "Chemo brain" (at least I have an excuse now).
- Hormonal treatment with tamoxifen puts you at risk for endometrial cancer and blood clots. Other hormonal treatments may be necessary for up to 10 years to block estrogen in the body, which may feed cancer if your cancer is estrogen positive.

Grieving the Losses and Moving on

I don't think it's hard to understand after reading that depressing list that many breast cancer patients take antidepressants. The changes in lifestyle, losses and medical issues can be overwhelming. For me, the losses I grieve are many, but a short list would include the loss of my breast, my health, the belief that I'll live to be a spry 100 year old, the temporary loss of lifestyle that makes me feel so good, the loss of natural bone density and muscle, the loss of the appearance of youth and the possible loss of my heart health.

Physically, I can do a lot to feel I have some control. Weight gain of more than 12 pounds puts me at higher risk of mortality, so eating and exercise have never been more important. It just requires finding the days when I have the most energy to do what I can and accepting those when I can't. It might not mean working out like I'm used to, but it's accepting that walking for 10 minutes is better than not walking. I can lessen the muscle and bone loss by doing strength training and lessen future injuries and joint problems.

The human spirit is incredible. We can take a lot and get up each day with a renewed spirit no matter what life throw us. It might take time, but we can heal. The primary motivation is that life is good, really. I savor each day and moment that I feel good. I savor time with friends and family and when I can make a contribution world, no matter how small. The one cancer can't do is take away my spirit. I am still me, through it all.

The Gifts and the Light

Is there a bright side to cancer? Unless you really are a pessimist at heart, it would be hard not to find some light. The compassion and kindness found in every walk of life, from strangers to acquaintances to relatives and friends is amazing. The humanity is comforting and healing. Because I've always been very independent, accepting support from others has been a challenge. I've gotten a lot better, but I have remembered words of wisdom from a fellow coach who told me that I was giving a gift to the giver when I allowed them to help me.

There are gifts like my college roommate flying out from Texas to be with me on my first day of chemo. Or the special portrait that captured my "feminine beauty" (their words) before the surgery and chemo began from a close friend and her sister, a portrait artist in Hilton Head. Or the canned wild salmon from the northwest to nourish me from a colleague and friend. The gifts of food that people take time to put together amidst their busy lives amaze me most. But what means more than any material gift is the gift of friendship and love from family and friends that I've been so blessed with.

My friend who passed away left a beautiful group of women who have become my close friends. I don't know how I'd be doing without them.

The opportunities for deepened relationships with family and friends are no doubt a gift. My boys are my personal trainers. Jeremy, my 20 year old, gets up early before work/school a few days a week to help me when I don't feel like going to do my strength training, and Dustin, my 18 year old, walks with me. My husband even helps with my daily shots.

The opportunities and coincidences because of the disease have been unique. From meeting a Harvard breast surgeon dealing with breast cancer at the ACSM conference the first week of my diagnosis to the plane trip back home, sitting beside a woman and her Duke physician husband, who was a few years past her breast cancer treatment at Duke. They were gifts of information for me I really needed at the time.

I've been blessed with great doctors and their staffs. My breast surgeon, Dr. Lee Wilke, immediately saw me as the individual I am and has helped me through some rough times. She, as all my doctors and their staffs, has been patient with my need for information and research, as well as offering great compassion.

I know I am not going through this alone. My family's lives have been changed forever. I am so grateful for every relationship I have, no matter how big or small, as they all bring something wonderful to my life. Through the giving I've received, I have learned how to better reach out to others who are hurting.

At the end of the day, I know that there is great suffering in this world and my problems are not that bad. I have so much to be thankful for. So for today, I feel good and I feel blessed.

About the Author

Pam Schmid received her B.S. in education/special education from the University of Texas at Austin with a psychology minor. She has been a health and fitness professional in the area of health promotion and disease prevention since 1981, holding numerous positions and certifications, including ACSM Health Fitness Specialist, ACSM's Cancer Exercise Trainer, and Wellcoaches Wellness Coaching certification.

After her diagnosis of breast cancer in 2004, Pam began speaking and writing to educate and empower patients. Her business, Priorities Simplified, provides wellness services, including wellness coaching, speaking and consulting, to individuals, businesses, and organizations. She has served as teaching faculty at Wellcoaches Corporation since 2003.

She is the creator of Healthy and Fit After Cancer® programs, which were established to give survivors a pathway to feeling their best with powerful, yet practical steps that inspire hope, possibility, and strength to follow their vision of health and well-being after a diagnosis of cancer.

Pam is an international speaker, coach, and writer who has been interviewed and quoted by local, national, and international media, including *USA Today*, *U.S. News & World Report*, *USA Today*, CBN, and ABC and CBS local. She has been a patient advocate at the local, state, and national levels for several organizations, was a founding member of the Duke Patient Advocacy Council, co-chair for the North Carolina Comprehensive Cancer Survivorship Workgroup, and three-time Lance Armstrong Foundation LIVE**STRONG** national delegate, Global Summit volunteer, and LIVE**STRONG** leader. She was also the recipient of the Jonquil Award in 2005, from the Duke University Comprehensive Cancer Center. Schmid is currently featured in the national public service announcements reaching more than 100 million people in the Mammography Saves Lives campaign (mammographysaveslives.org).

Pam and Jerry, her husband of over 30 years, have two grown boys, Jeremy and Dustin, and a new daughter-in-law, Caroline. She enjoys acting and has been in numerous commercials, films, and corporate videos.